first-time mom's pregnancy activity book

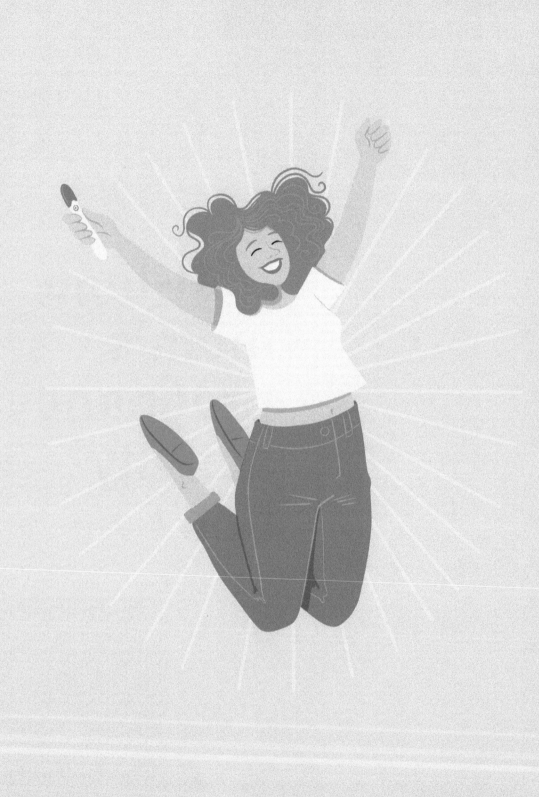

first-time mom's pregnancy activity book

100 FUN GAMES,
PROJECTS, AND PROMPTS TO
PREPARE FOR BABY

Tabitha Blue

Illustrations by Amy Blackwell

ROCKRIDGE
PRESS

Interior and Cover Designer: Lisa Forde
Art Producer: Samantha Ulban
Editor: Shannon Criss
Production Editor: Emily Sheehan

Illustrations by © 2020 Amy Blackwell.
Author Photo Courtesy of © Briony Skerjance.

ISBN: Print 978-1-64611-948-6

R0

To my favorite people on this side of Heaven:
Chris, Aliyah, Brayden, Skylar, Aria, Lennon,
and Quinn. And to our two in Heaven.

I've experienced it all with you; the learning,
the growing, the stretching, the new life together.
I'm a mother because of all of you.

Contents

Second Trimester (13 to 28 Weeks)

Third Trimester (28 to 40 Weeks)

Childbirth

Letter to Moms

Dear New Mom,

Congratulations! You're starting one of the most exciting chapters of your life. Whether you've received the news of your pregnancy with excitement or trepidation, one thing is certain: There is a heart beating near your own, and it's the beginning of a bond like you've never known.

I remember when it came time to deliver my first born. I wasn't ready. While many people around me were hoping I'd deliver on my due date, I wished for more time. Now, with six kids (and after recently giving birth to twins), I've experienced a wide range of different pregnancies and births. So, Mama, you've got this! You might have a lot of questions or feel a little overwhelmed, but both are typical experiences of a first-time mom. Good news—this book is here to help in a really fun way.

The following pages are filled with relevant exercises and activities to help you prepare for the arrival of your little one. I encourage you to use this book as your own personal guide and journal equipped with plenty of space for your thoughts and feelings.

The activities are divided into four sections: First Trimester, Second Trimester, Third Trimester, and Childbirth. But I want you to digest it all in a way that is most comfortable for you. Skip around. Jump from section to section. Write notes in the margin, and highlight things you plan to revisit. Use this book as you please, especially during downtime, on those nights you can't sleep, or while nesting. And, most importantly, dismiss judgments from others as you make decisions and cherish this time spent preparing for the sweet pea growing inside of you.

Welcome to Motherhood,
Tabitha Blue

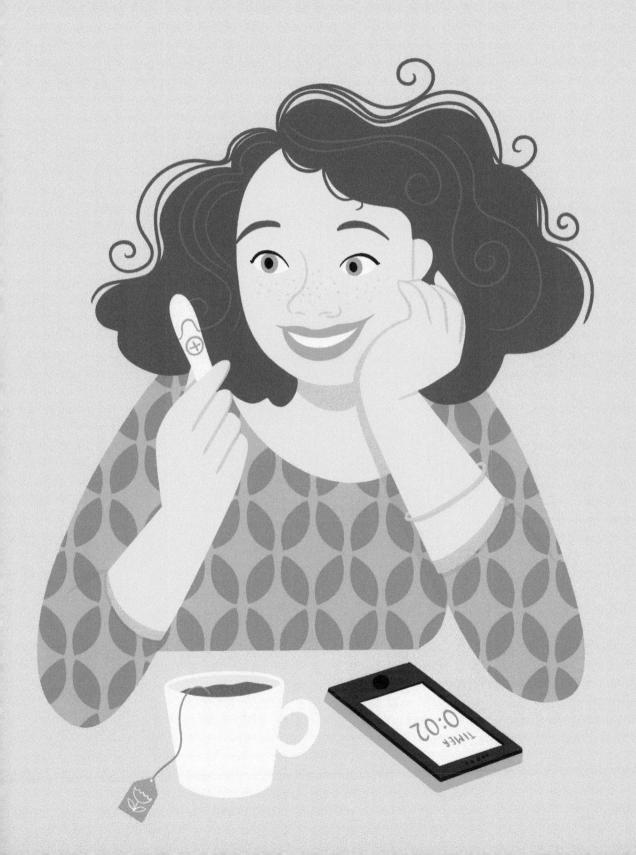

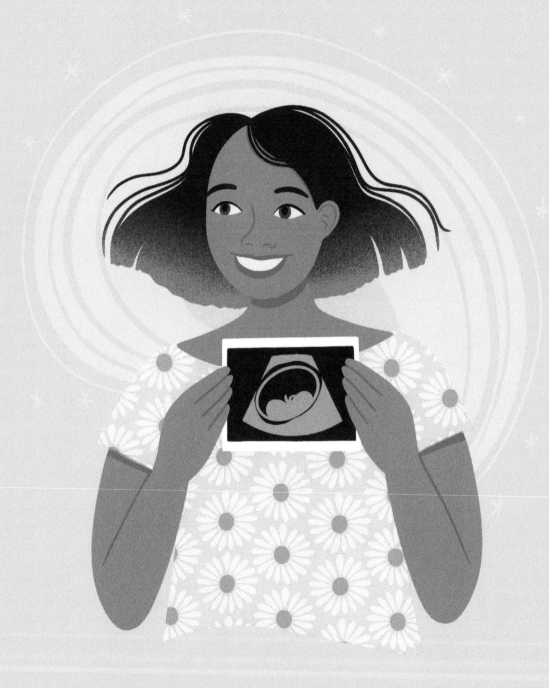

First Trimester

(1 TO 13 WEEKS)

Amazing Mama

Help guide this pregnant mama to the hospital for her first appointment.

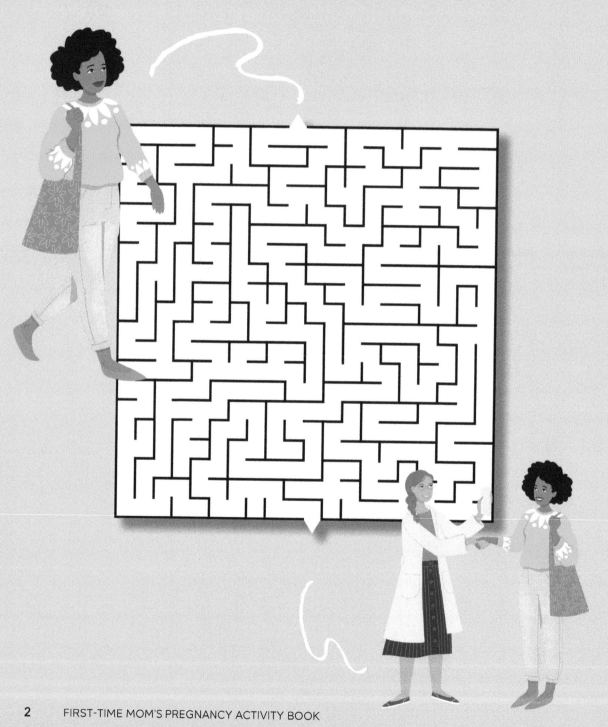

Due Date Calculator

The average pregnancy lasts around 40 weeks, but a due date is just an estimation. Babies come when they're ready! If you are ready to estimate your due date, simply count 40 weeks, or 280 days, from the first day of your last menstrual period.

What was the FIRST day of your last period? _____

Now subtract THREE months: _____

Then add SEVEN days: _____

(For example, if your last period started on January 1, you'd count back three months to October 1 and then add seven days, which means your due date would be October 8!)

Remember: Your due date is an estimate. It's completely normal and safe to deliver between 38 and 42 weeks, so don't be surprised if you go into labor a week or two before or after your EDD (estimated due date). The percentage of women who deliver on their due date is extremely low. If you know the exact date of conception, your EDD will be 38 weeks from that day.

What excites you about your due date? _____

_____

_____

_____

What is your favorite part of that season? _____

_____

_____

_____

Selecting Your Hospital and Doctor Checklist

Asking friends or family for recommendations is helpful and valid when it comes to medical decisions, but this choice is also very personal, and you may find that what worked for someone else doesn't work for you. Finding a doctor and a hospital that align with your own birth philosophy is what's important.

For example, if you want a natural birth, you'll need to find a hospital that will support skipping an epidural. If you're experiencing a high-risk pregnancy, you'll want a hospital with specialized care and NICU (neonatal intensive care unit) services available for your baby.

Over the next couple of weeks, work your way through this checklist for selecting the best doctor and hospital for you!

☐ **Check with your insurance.** It's time to look at what coverage you have and get a list of which hospitals, doctors, and midwives are considered "in network" and are covered by your insurance. Going out of network can be costly.

☐ **Figure out what kind of care are you looking for.** Circle one: Doctor/OB-GYN or Midwife

☐ **Get recommendations from friends or family.** If those providers are in network, start there.

☐ **Consider your health history.** If you've experienced previous pregnancy complications or other health issues, you may need to look into a maternal-fetal medicine practice that can provide high-risk obstetric care.

Questions to ask the OB-GYN or midwife you're considering:

☐ How long have they been practicing?

☐ How often will you see them before and after childbirth?

☐ What options do they recommend for pain management?

- ☐ How do they handle complications?

- ☐ Do they provide support throughout the labor?

- ☐ Where are their admitting privileges (at which hospitals can they deliver)?

- ☐ Lastly, it's important to go with your gut. Do you feel comfortable with the OB-GYN?

Once you find a doctor or midwife you're comfortable with, during your appointment, ask for their advice about hospitals. They will know the level of care you and your baby will need, and they'll usually know a lot about the hospitals in your area.

Questions to answer about the hospital you're considering:

- ☐ How far is it from home? How long does it take to get there? (Remember, you may be in labor and need to get there quickly!)

- ☐ Does it support my preferred delivery method (vaginal, C-section, or unmedicated)?

- ☐ What level of NICU care does the hospital provide?

- ☐ What kind of prenatal education classes are offered?

- ☐ What type of care and lactation support are offered after birth?

- ☐ What is the nurse to patient ratio?

- ☐ Are private rooms available?

- ☐ What are the rules about visitors?

Finally, schedule a tour of the hospital where you'd like to deliver to make sure that you feel comfortable and that getting there is easy.

Growing Baby

Growing a baby is hard work, but coloring one isn't!

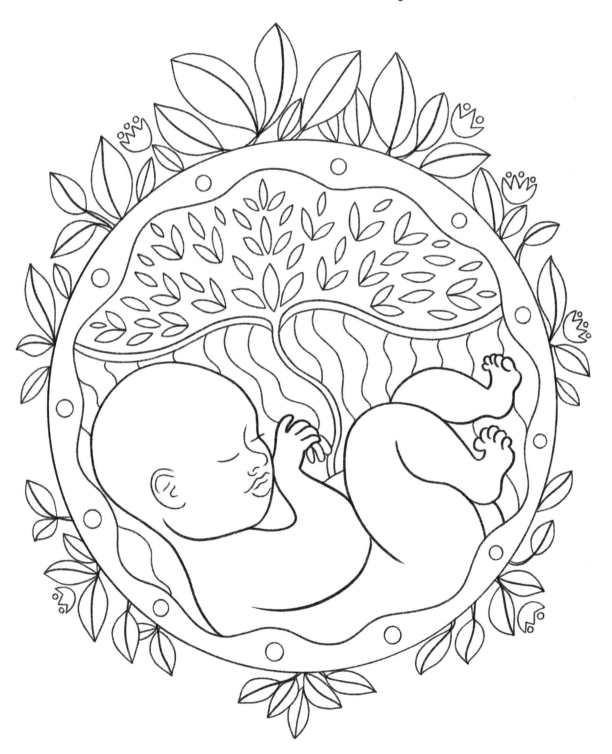

Gestation Indications

Sometimes these symptoms are the first sign of pregnancy! Find and circle the pregnancy symptoms in the grid. Look for them in all directions, including backward and diagonally.

Fatigue

Nausea

Vomiting

Food aversions

Food cravings

Lower back pain

Tender breasts

Bloating

Flatulence

Mood swings

Vaginal discharge

Skin changes

Dizziness

Headaches

Constipation

Frequent urination

Light spotting

```
B L O A T I N G H E A D A C H E S E N Q
S K I N C H A N G E S E C X F O C U S R
N D M N O I T A N I R U Z Y M S F G S O
O C E I N P E D O O C E D A E R P I E U
I T G Z F L A T U L E N C E Z L E T N G
T E R N B E G E R E O I V C A N E A I N
A N A M X F O O D C R A V I N G S F Z I
P D H S C L I G H T S P O T T I N G Z T
I E C B G G A N D E T K D N O A Y O I I
T R S P F N M N P P A C A E S U A N D M
S B I S N O I S R E V A D O O F Y E F O
N R D E T I B W A P N B V B R E D Y T V
O E P P U I T Y S M M R W Q A K C W T E
C A M D Y X U P T D A E H V U E U U F A
E S V A G I N A L A O W T N E U Q E R F
N T A J W I Y P F N V O O J I E E P U Q
M S B G J M E C V T U L M K I I N Z M G
```

9 TIPS TO EASE MORNING SICKNESS

1. **Stay hydrated.** It's crucial to stay hydrated, and if you can't keep fluids down, try letting ice melt in your mouth. Drink 30 minutes before and after meals, but not during them.

2. **Don't let your stomach get empty.** Keep bland snacks like crackers on your nightstand. Nibble them first thing in the morning to get a little something on your stomach before you even sit up all the way.

3. **Try a bland diet.** High-protein and low-fat foods or mild foods like bananas may be easier for you to digest. If you're looking for something to sip, ginger, peppermint, or fennel tea can be super soothing to a sour stomach.

4. **Get on your feet.** Go for a walk or find other ways to move to get your blood circulating. This will help balance hormones and in turn ease your morning sickness.

5. **Use aromatherapy.** There are some scents that can ease morning sickness, like lemon, ginger, orange, and mint. Instead of using a room spray, add a drop or two of your favorite scent to a cotton ball to place under your nose so that if the scent doesn't sit well with you, you can easily remove it.

6. **Try a lollipop.** Grab some pregnancy lollipops or ginger candies. Both can help alleviate morning sickness.

7. **Avoid strong smells.** Steer clear of scents likely to trigger you. For many, those triggers are things like cigarette smoke, strong coffee, meat cooking (open the windows or ask someone else to do the cooking), and perfumes.

8. **Take your vitamins.** Many doctors recommend B6 for easing nausea symptoms. See if your prenatal vitamins have this, and ask about taking extra B vitamins as well, especially if you're having trouble keeping the multivitamin down.

9. **Medication.** If morning sickness is extreme for you and you've tried everything else, talk to your doctor about safe medications for nausea.

PREGNANCY SYMPTOMS 101

No matter where you are in your pregnancy journey, your emotions can be a roller coaster, especially during the first trimester when your hormones are soaring.

These feelings are all completely normal. You're not alone in having them or in having mood swings. Give yourself grace, take care of yourself, rest, and look to family members for understanding during this time of change.

The following are a few completely normal pregnancy symptoms you may experience in the first trimester:

Swollen or tender breasts: As your body adjusts to the hormone changes, you'll see this level off.

Headaches: Headaches can be a side effect of increased hormones and blood volume. Staying hydrated, getting enough sleep, and reducing stress are all ways to help prevent this symptom. Using a warm or cold compress can help with reducing the pain.

Heartburn: During pregnancy, progesterone helps "relax" your body. Unfortunately, this process also relaxes the valve between your stomach and esophagus, causing heartburn. Best way to help avoid it? Steer clear of spicy or acidic foods.

Constipation: Back to those hormones again! Between increased hormones and iron supplements in your prenatal vitamin, constipation is a very common pregnancy symptom. Drinking plenty of fluids and eating high-fiber foods can help.

Fatigue: The hormone progesterone kicks into high gear in the first trimester, which can make you feel sleepy. Get rest when you can. Your body is working really hard, even if you can't quite tell yet. Light physical activity can give you a boost of energy as well.

Frequent urination: Hormonal changes will make you pee more. You'll see this decrease after the first trimester—and then pick up again in the third trimester once your baby is larger and putting increased pressure on your bladder.

From Fear to Excitement

Whenever we're heading into something new, it's completely normal to feel uneasy. Pregnancy is no different. It's natural to worry about the unknown.

So, Mama, when those feelings come up, understand that it's normal. You are strong, so many women have been exactly where you are, and you, too, can get through this.

Think about a time in your life when you were brave, and fill in the blanks, keeping in mind what brave looks like right now.

I am strong because: _____

_____

I am brave because: _____

_____

I love being pregnant because: _____

_____

I am excited because: _____

_____

The first time I hear my baby's heartbeat I will feel: _____

_____

I like to imagine life with my baby because: _____

_____

I am beautiful because: _____

_____

I am most looking forward to: _____

_____

The Association of Motherhood

Look at the word **MOTHERHOOD**. Then, at the end of each line radiating from **MOTHERHOOD**, quickly write down the first word that comes to mind. Try not to pause or think too much. When you're finished, reflect on what you wrote.

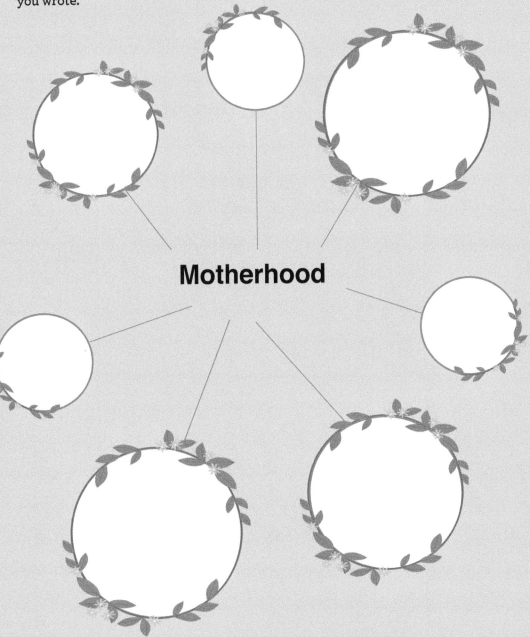

Motherhood

Foods to Avoid

While pregnancy brings certain dietary perks—hello, perfect excuse to eat that last bite!—there are a few foods you will need to leave off the table until after your baby is born. Answer the clues in the crossword puzzle to find out what foods should be avoided during pregnancy.

Across

3. Spread-able dairy
5. Jolt of energy you crave in a cup of Joe
7. Udder to table milk
8. Raw
9. Hot flavor
10. Cold cuts

Down

1. Japanese bar fare
2. Edible trash
4. Lofty planet
6. Sweet drink sold in cartons

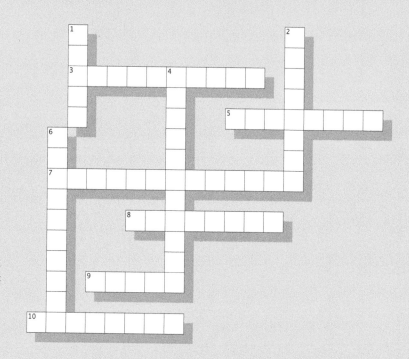

PREGNANCY DIET NO-NOS

Your body is already experiencing many changes and working overtime during a pregnancy, especially in the first trimester. You want to eat right when you're expecting, and trying to figure out what that means can sometimes feel overwhelming. Besides taking prenatal vitamins, getting enough water, and adding in a few extra calories (about 300 extra calories a day is all you need), there's the subject of what not to eat.

You're in the season of dreaming of your sweet babe, but it's also a season of a weakened immune system. During pregnancy, you're more susceptible to outside organisms like bacteria, viruses, and other pollutants that can cause foodborne illnesses.

Also, since you're sharing just about everything with your unborn baby, that goes for what you eat as well. Anything you ingest is likely to cross the placenta, so it's imperative to be careful with what you eat, as well as how you handle food. With that said, there are a few foods that expecting mamas should steer clear of, both for your own health and safety as well as for your baby.

The list of foods to avoid mainly consists of undercooked or unpasteurized foods, which are more likely to carry bacteria and parasites that haven't been killed off in the cooking or heating process.

Along with safe food handling, like washing your hands often, it's also a good idea to clean out the refrigerator regularly and make sure food is fully cooked. In fact, that's first on the list of foods to avoid—raw or undercooked food (including fish, meat, and eggs). Save sushi for a postpartum celebration!

You'll also need to stay away from unpasteurized foods, which include some types of cheese, milk, deli meats, and juices. Fish with high mercury levels, like tuna, aren't a good idea either. And we can't forget about drinks! While caffeine is okay in small amounts (about 200 milligrams of caffeine or less a day, which is about 12 ounces of coffee), it's recommended to steer clear of alcohol for the time being.

Don't worry, though, there's an upside! Besides keeping your baby safe, this food avoidance won't last forever—there are still plenty of foods to eat . . . and plenty you *should* eat.

PREGNANCY KEY NUTRIENTS

Now that we know what not to eat, I'm sure you're wondering what you should eat.

Well, everything else is still on the table! You should focus especially on getting your calcium, iron, and folate.

A good prenatal vitamin is a great place to start and will give you a boost of vitamins and minerals. If your stomach can handle it, ask your doctor about a prenatal vitamin with added iron as it's one of the nutrients that is often lacking during pregnancy.

Iron makes up a major portion of hemoglobin, found in red blood cells, and is what carries oxygen throughout the body. By the end of your pregnancy, your body will have up to 60 percent more blood than usual, which means you need more iron to keep up with that level of blood production. Iron can be hard on the stomach, so if you're feeling strong morning sickness, you may need to wait until after it subsides. Thankfully, there are plenty of foods that contain iron, like whole grains, dark green vegetables, and lean meat.

Additionally, the CDC recommends that you take 400 micrograms of folic acid every day. Folic acid, or folate, is a key vitamin that decreases the risk of neural tube defects. Basically a superhero for your baby's developing brain, this B vitamin is easy to add into your daily routine. So, look into a folic acid supplement, and have a bite of your favorite green salad or fortified cereal, too!

Since your body doesn't produce calcium, and it's needed for the strong bones and teeth that are being developed in your uterus, you need 1,000 milligrams of calcium daily. You can get it by noshing on spinach, kale, and dairy products, or by adding in a supplement.

Why is it important to add in the right amounts of these vitamins and minerals? Your body wants to ensure a healthy fetus and will get as many of the nutrients that it needs for your growing baby from your own body, meaning you'll start to become deficient if you're not adding in additional foods or supplements to supply these needs.

Don't overthink it, though. The biggest thing to remember about what you eat is to listen to your body, and also to take a prenatal vitamin!

The Most Essential Glass

Connect the dots to reveal one of the most
essentials liquids during pregnancy.

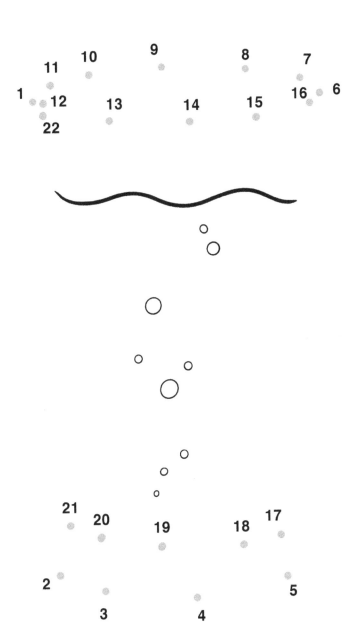

H2O DURING PREGNANCY

It's time to raise a glass to celebrate your pregnancy! A glass of clean, pure water, that is.

The American Pregnancy Association recommends 8 to 12 glasses of water daily, with an additional glass for every hour of light exercise. How do you know that you're getting enough: Your urine is pale and you're urinating often!

So, let's dive into these benefits.

- Staying properly hydrated can help prevent urinary tract infections, constipation, and hemorrhoids, all of which are common pregnancy issues.
- H_2O helps you feel better! Some women notice that drinking more water helps keep morning sickness, heartburn, and indigestion at bay. Even more so, dehydration is a main cause of headaches, dizziness, and cramping. Avoid these pains—literally—with adequate water intake.
- Water not only helps deliver vitamins, nutrients, oxygen, and hormones throughout your body, it's also the key for making sure these essential properties reach your baby through the placenta.
- Feeling fatigued? Try drinking more water. It helps keep that fatigue in check.
- Water helps rid the body of excess sodium and reduces water retention, a common symptom during pregnancy. In turn, this helps reduce swelling in your ankles.

Tip: If you're having trouble keeping water down during the first trimester morning sickness, keep ice chips handy.

So, bottoms up, Mama.

Pregnancy Exercises Quiz

Now that you're growing a human being inside your body, you may be wondering whether you should be jostling yourself around with exercise. Take this quiz to see how much you know about working out with a bun in the oven.

1. **Is it safe to exercise during pregnancy?**

   A. Yes, of course!

   B. You may want to wait for a little while before engaging in physical activity.

   C. No, exercise is bad!

   D. Does putting on my shoes count?

2. **You can keep doing most of the exercises you did before you were pregnant.**

   T / F

3. **I love my ab workout. When should I stop doing ab exercises during my pregnancy?**

   A. First Trimester

   B. Second Trimester

   C. Third Trimester

   D. Talk to your doctor about your routine to figure out what's safe.

4. **Which exercise may be beneficial during your delivery?**

   A. Squats

   B. Scissor Legs

   C. Sipping Coffee

   D. Kegels

5. **What should be a priority when exercising during pregnancy?**

   A. Orthopedic shoes

   B. Supportive bra

   C. Updated playlist

   D. Maternity belt

6. **Why do doctors recommend swimming as a particularly safe exercise?**

   A. The humidity eases morning sickness.

   B. The water relieves tender breasts.

   C. You can't fall while in the water.

   D. The smell is invigorating.

7. **I'm planning a babymoon before I give birth. What water sport should I avoid?**

   A. Snorkeling

   B. Water aerobics

   C. Scuba diving

   D. Wading

8. **Contact sports are okay for pregnant women, as long as they're very careful.**

   T / F

9. **Which style of yoga should be avoided during pregnancy?**

   A. Hatha

   B. Bikram

   C. Iyengar

   D. Ashtanga

10. **How many extra calories should I eat per day during pregnancy?**

    A. 100

    B. 300

    C. 500

    D. 1,000

11. **If you experience _____ during exercise, you should immediately stop.**

    A. Headache or dizziness

    B. Abdominal pain/contraction

    C. Chest pain

    D. All of the above

THE RULES OF EXERCISE WHILE PREGNANT

Though you may only feel like sleeping in the first trimester, there are quite a few benefits to exercise and physical activity throughout your pregnancy, including reduced fatigue. In fact, exercise during pregnancy can help reduce back pain and stress and increase stamina (which you'll need for labor and delivery). It also decreases the risk for some of the more serious potential complications of pregnancy and birth, like gestational diabetes and preeclampsia.

Just start slow! It's not time to set up a new exercise routine by trying to run a marathon. If you've already had certain physical activities as part of a normal routine, you should be able to keep up with those. Adding in physical activity doesn't mean introducing a big, new routine, but daily walks and low-impact exercises like swimming are recommended for pregnancy.

So how much exercise do you need? Unless you have a medical issue or pregnancy complication, it's been recommended by the American College of Obstetrics and Gynecology to engage in moderate exercise for at least 20 to 30 minutes a day most or all days of the week. Sometimes this is simply deciding to *move* every day. It might be a stroll through the mall, stretches on the yoga mat while you catch up on your favorite show, or marching in place while you cook dinner. Either way, make sure to listen to your body, take breaks when you need to, and stay hydrated!

Let's talk about what precautions you should take in setting up a successful exercise routine.

- Drink plenty of water beforehand and throughout your physical activity. Dehydration is never something you want to deal with, but it's even more imperative to stay hydrated during pregnancy.
- Invest in a good, supportive bra! A great bra will be your best friend, especially during physical activity. Your breasts can be sensitive and swollen, but the right bra can help ensure a more comfortable workout.
- Avoid lying flat on your back as this can limit blood flow to your baby. This means finding alternatives for exercises like crunches, etc.
- Swimming exercises are safe, pressure-relieving ways to get your blood flowing. Just avoid scuba diving as it can put you at risk for "bends," allowing for harmful air bubbles in the baby's blood vessels.
- Avoid overheating. Stay cool by exercising in an air-conditioned room or do outdoor activities during the cooler hours of the day.

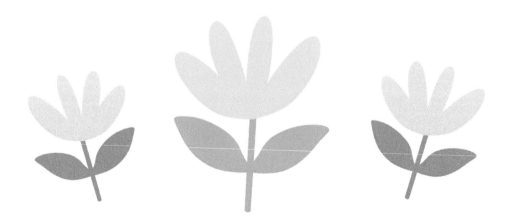

Pregnancy Moods

The first trimester brings along so many changes! Fill in the blanks to track how you're feeling during these first 12 weeks of pregnancy.

I am craving _____

_____

I am avoiding _____

_____

I am feeling _____

_____

I am excited about _____

_____

I am reading _____

_____

I am watching _____

_____

I am thinking about _____

_____

I am most nervous about _____

_____

I am laughing because _____

_____

I am happy about _____

_____

PET SAFETY AND PREGNANCY

One of the biggest questions when you're already a mama to fur babies is whether pets pose a risk to your baby. The long and short answer is yes, pets *can* pose a health risk. The great news is that there are precautions you can take so that you, your baby, and your pets stay healthy and happy. And NO, you don't have to get rid of your furry babies, banish them to the great outdoors, or limit your interaction with them.

The health concern that is most associated with pets when it comes to pregnancy is toxoplasmosis, a parasite that animals can carry and excrete in their feces. This is especially of concern with indoor cats, since you're more likely to come in contact with feces as you clean the litter box. The easy solution here? Put someone else on daily litter box duty when you're pregnant! If that's not an option, you can wear gloves and wash your hands thoroughly as preventive measures.

We also aren't sure of the effects of veterinary medications, like heartworm or flea and tick medicines, on an unborn baby. If your pet needs topical medication, wear gloves during application and wash your hands thoroughly after or let someone else take over flea meds duty.

If you're already thinking about preparing your pets for your baby's arrival, there are some things you can consider, like obedience classes, if your dog hasn't had them before. It might sound crazy, but having a baby doll around the house can be a good way to prep your animal for another little guest. Practice holding the doll, placing it in the crib, holding it to rock, setting it in the stroller . . . and start to train your pet to stay out of the crib or bassinet.

Finally, slowly adjust the amount of time and attention you're giving your fur babies instead of an immediate withdrawal once your focus is on taking care of the baby. Luckily, babies don't move around much on their own for at least six months, so your pet will have some time to get used to your child before things get really tricky. The biggest challenge you'll face is when your little baby is excited to crawl everywhere and grab everything—including your fur baby!

First Trimester Firsts

Unscramble the words for an idea of what firsts to expect in the first trimester.

kkci __ __ __ __

udnuoatrls __ __ __ __ __ __ __ __ __ __

rootdc __ __ __ __ __ __

tteehrbaa __ __ __ __ __ __ __ __ __

snaaue __ __ __ __ __ __

stuef __ __ __ __ __

gvrcian __ __ __ __ __ __ __

nsehmoro __ __ __ __ __ __ __ __

detir __ __ __ __ __

gmnrion sesskcin __ __ __ __ __ __ __ __ __ __ __ __

domo wgniss __ __ __ __ __ __ __ __ __ __

gtwieh angi __ __ __ __ __ __ __ __ __ __

tlpanare __ __ __ __ __ __ __ __

eetcign ttsse __ __ __ __ __ __ __ __ __ __ __

yabb esmna __ __ __ __ __ __ __ __ __

sntlieas __ __ __ __ __ __ __ __

sett __ __ __ __

eevltw kesew __ __ __ __ __ __ __ __ __ __ __

naevrsio __ __ __ __ __ __ __ __

First Trimester Quiz

Test your pregnancy knowledge of the things you need to know during your first trimester.

1. **Which hormone gives the pregnancy test a positive readout?**
   A. HCG
   B. Testosterone
   C. Estrogen
   D. Progesterone

2. **Experiencing heartburn during the first trimester may be evidence that your baby will have a full head of hair.**

   T / F

3. **Nearly 1 in 3 women will most likely give birth in this manner.**
   A. Vaginally, with no drugs
   B. Via surrogate
   C. C-section
   D. At home

4. **What does "in utero" mean?**
   A. Bank owed
   B. Algae found in deepest part of ocean
   C. In the uterus
   D. Incomprehensible

5. **While a high percentage of babies are born *after* their due date, what percentage come on the actual due date?**
   A. Around 5 percent
   B. Around 10 percent
   C. Around 15 percent
   D. More than 20 percent

6. **What sleeping position do most doctors recommend?**
   A. Back
   B. Right side
   C. Stomach
   D. Left side

7. **Listeria is a bacteria found in certain foods that may be harmful to baby. What is a food you could find listeria in?**
   A. Unwashed fruit/veggies
   B. Undercooked meat and seafood
   C. Unpasteurized cheeses and milk
   D. All of the above

8. **Good dental hygiene helps during pregnancy because changes in hormones can lead to...**

    A. Gingivitis

    B. Loose teeth

    C. Bad breath

    D. Both A and B

9. **Toxoplasmosis is a mild infection that a mother can pass to her unborn baby. The infection can be associated with what?**

    A. Exposure to cat feces

    B. Consuming undercooked or contaminated meat

    C. Drinking whole milk

    D. Both A and B

10. **Doctors recommend avoiding use of topical skin care with this ingredient because it may be bad for your baby.**

    A. Retinoid

    B. Skin-lightening cream

    C. Neither A nor B

    D. Both A and B

11. **It's safe to get an X-ray while pregnant.**

    True or False

12. **Omega-3 fatty acids are good for baby's brain and eye development. What is a good amount to consume daily?**

    A. 300 mg

    B. 1000 mg

    C. 100 mg

    D. 12 oz

13. **It's possible to take too many vitamins.**

    T / F

14. **What percentage of women will experience morning sickness?**

    A. 10 percent

    B. 25 percent

    C. 50 percent

    D. 75 percent

Out of Order

These stages of pregnancy are out of chronological order. See if you can figure out the week when your pregnancy might be reaching each developmental milestone. This is a fun way to see how your baby is progressing and growing, even when you may not see your bump yet.

The first is done as an example.
1 week - Period

_____ Genitals start to form

_____ Ovulation

_____ Baby's heart begins to form

_____ Toes start to form

_____ Fingers begin to form

_____ Buds appear that will become arms

_____ Implantation

_____ Head develops

_____ Fertilization

_____ Elbows can bend

Spread the News!

You've most likely already thought about how you want to announce your exciting news. Some women spill the beans to friends, family, and coworkers right away. Some like to shout it from the rooftops by spreading the news on social media as soon as they find out. Others wait until they're in their second trimester, when their pregnancy is well established and the *risk of miscarriage* has declined significantly.

Deciding how and when to share the news is a personal decision and completely up to you: There's no wrong choice. Don't put added pressure on yourself to do or say anything that you aren't comfortable with. You can choose to savor this as a sweet little secret, or you can celebrate the news by sharing it early.

So, how do you want to announce your pregnancy?

If you're still on the fence, we've got a few ideas that might get your creativity flowing!

- **Baby shoes.** Who can resist mini footwear lined up next to your own?

- **Chalk.** Writing out a cheeky announcement phrase in chalk is a fun option.

- **Letterboard.** Get on trend with this fun photo addition. It's a great way to share the month you're expecting a new arrival.

- **Beach.** Live near the water? Write your announcement in the sand!

- **Onesie.** These tiny outfits are a cute way to show off the fact that you've got a baby on the way.

- **Clothing.** Create T-shirts, jerseys, or jackets with words like "mama" on the back. Wear it proud!

HERE WE GO, EMBRYO

With all the changes happening in your body, it's fun to learn about what is happening in your baby's body as well.

Though pregnancy symptoms can start early on, it'll be quite a while before you feel baby move. But even before you see those lines on the pregnancy stick, your body is hard at work!

Because your due date is calculated at 40 weeks from the first day of your last period, during the first two weeks of your official pregnancy, you're not even pregnant yet. Those first two weeks are when your period takes place and your body is preparing for pregnancy. It's not until the end of your second week and sometimes even into your third week that ovulation and conception occur. As it moves through your fallopian tube, your fertilized egg divides into more cells. Once these cells make it to your uterus, they float around in a ball for a few days. When that ball of cells attaches to your uterus, that's called implantation—it happens around week 3 or 4. This is when you're actually pregnant, and it's also when your embryo starts developing its first nerve cells.

By week 7, though your baby is less than an inch long and you're not showing yet (besides the swollen breasts and what might feel like bloat), your baby has webbed fingers and toes and a heart. This is usually when your first prenatal visit will happen, as most doctors like to schedule it between 6 and 8 weeks.

At the end of your third month of pregnancy, also the end of your first trimester, external genitals have developed, and all vital organs and extremities from the ears to the toes are forming. By that time, your baby is about two and a half inches long!

Whew, that was a busy trimester!

First Trimester Checklist

All the chores that need to be completed from your first pregnancy test to holding your baby in your arms can feel overwhelming; take it one trimester at a time! Here are items you can focus on in the first 12 weeks.

- ☐ Take a pregnancy test.
- ☐ Tell your partner the good news.
- ☐ Check your health insurance policy to see what prenatal and childbirth care is covered.
- ☐ Find an OB-GYN or other prenatal care provider.
- ☐ Schedule your first prenatal checkup.
- ☐ If you currently smoke, quit.
- ☐ Avoid drinking alcohol.
- ☐ Make sure your exercise is pregnancy-safe.
- ☐ Begin taking prenatal vitamins, including folic acid supplements.
- ☐ Start avoiding hazardous foods.
- ☐ Figure out how pregnancy, maternity leave, and a new baby will affect your finances.

- ☐ Go to your first prenatal checkup (right around week 8).
- ☐ Consult your provider about medications you're taking.
- ☐ Consider doing a first trimester screening to determine the risk of chromosomal abnormalities between weeks 11 and 14.
- ☐ Decide whether or not you'd like to learn the sex of the baby.
- ☐ Start taking weekly pregnancy photos.
- ☐ Research the maternity leave policy at your workplace.
- ☐ Start a baby name list.
- ☐ Look into childbirth classes.
- ☐ Rest!

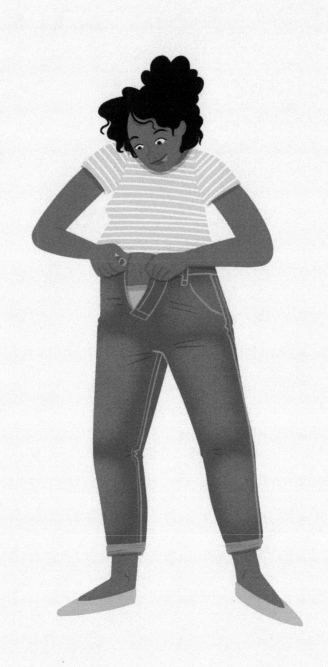

Second Trimester

(13 TO 28 WEEKS)

What Size Is My Baby?

Draw a line to match the food with the size of the baby throughout pregnancy, starting at 4 weeks, when the embryo has implanted in your uterus. Color in each fruit as your baby grows.

4 WEEKS - poppy seed

7 WEEKS - blueberry

9 WEEKS - grape

12 WEEKS - lime

16 WEEKS - avocado

18 WEEKS - bell pepper

22 WEEKS - coconut

27 WEEKS - sweet potato

33 WEEKS - pineapple

39 WEEKS - mini watermelon

40 WEEKS - small pumpkin

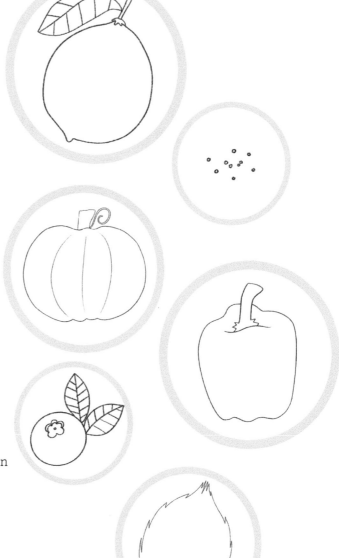

What to Expect When You're Expanding

Find and circle some of the completely normal changes you may experience in the second trimester. Look for them in all directions, including backward and diagonally.

Larger belly

Growing breasts

Vivid dreams

Braxton Hicks

Contractions

Linea nigra

Stretch marks

Stuffiness

Hair growth

Relief from nausea

Bleeding gums

Dizziness

Leg cramps

Energy

Baby movement

```
T S W I M I C Y D I Z Z I N E S S S P F T A W Y N M
M I F E D B V B A B Y M O V E M E N T J T J L U L O
W S I S I U A B Z A I I X M I E N E R G Y I B G M V
A P P X U P L A E S G X H P R O U E A Y N O U F C T
F V D N C P A A D U I I Y E K O O S Y E H R B X Y S
K S E D J I R U T X O E B Y S F M A A O A A U F Q T
S N O I T C A R T N O C S K C I H N O T X A R B R U
E V B U H T W O R G R I A H C B I P U D A L T Q T F
W U T J N U S S W E U R C E G G I C X R Y W Y C V F
C E R E Y I Z C L E C U V J R L X O I S C P R K I I
U U R H V F B E V I Q J M A Y L L E B R E G R A L N
T T S C K R G T G Q P X E U J H D E A T M B V E R E
O I J N U C V O F P G R O W I N G B R E A S T S S S
A M Y C R U I Z R Y W Z C S K M M I P O L A O I W S
H S E A E S U A N M O R F F E I L E R T U H D A U R
L V M D C U O S I I O W K F M T C O O U V T T T V G
Y P R G C Y B J J F O O I T U F N P Z D O B V C I A
S M Y E A T F E X N X O E P U B R Y O M R O N A J T
Q M A U Y O O V I X S R E W C I P D I E O V O Z E S
J A Y V D F P V I Y T U E S I A V I F T E A A U A W
R V I V I D D R E A M S B L E E D I N G G U M S E S
L I C Y O S K R A M H C T E R T S Y N Y K Z A T T D
H Z Y L N E G F P P E A Y H E F O H M S L Z F P Y E
```

BRAXTON HICKS VS. REAL CONTRACTIONS

Along with the beauty of your changing body and the miracle of growing life within you, there's another little thing that can sometimes occur in the second trimester—Braxton Hicks contractions.

It's good to know a little about what these contractions are so that you're prepared if you start to feel them. You can think of Braxton Hicks contractions (named after the doctor who first diagnosed them) as practice labor. Even though these contractions are uncomfortable and sometimes painful, you're getting a chance to practice for baby's arrival, which is actually a good thing!

There are a few tricks to discerning whether the contractions you're feeling are Braxton Hicks contractions or real labor.

A Matter of Real vs. Fake

- With all contractions, you'll notice a tightening of your abdomen, and this is where you'll feel Braxton Hicks as well. With labor-inducing contractions, tightening can be accompanied by pain in the lower abdomen, the lower back, and sometimes even the legs.
- Consistency is another factor to consider. Real contractions typically last from 30 to 60 seconds in length and occur regularly, increasing in frequency (for example, every 10 minutes, then every 8 then every 5 minutes and so on). Braxton Hicks contractions do not follow a pattern in either length or in frequency.
- If you begin to feel contractions and you can't tell if your body is heading into real labor, change positions, pee, or walk around and drink a glass of water. If you've had a busy day, rest or relax your body with a warm bath. These steps will often halt Braxton Hicks contractions, but they won't affect true labor.
- A pinkish vaginal discharge can occur a few days before labor. Noticeable changes in your baby's movement, continuous leaking of fluid, or if your water breaks (which can be anything from a gush to a slow trickling of fluid) can be indicators of true contractions as well.

It's always wise to contact your doctor or midwife if you're not sure what's going on. It never hurts to ask, even if it turns out to be a false alarm.

An Ultrasound Story for the Ages

Write down the first word that comes to mind when you read these parts of speech. Then read the story aloud using the words from your list. This activity is especially fun when played with a partner. Take turns asking for words to fill in the blanks!

NOUN 1 (object) _____   NOUN 2 (object) _____

ADJECTIVE 1 _____   NOUN 3 (object) _____

ADJECTIVE 2 _____   ADJECTIVE 4 _____

ADJECTIVE 3 _____   COLOR 1 _____

VERB 1 _____-ing   VERB 2 _____

I went to my first ultrasound wearing a _____. It proved very
                                              NOUN 1

_____. The doctor was quite _____ with his _____
   ADJECTIVE 1   ADJECTIVE 2   ADJECTIVE 3

gloves. He was _____ the wand on my belly, and it was lubed with
                      VERB 1

_____. My heart flipped when I saw the baby for the first time with my
   NOUN 2

own two eyes and a _____. I decided right there and then I would put
                          NOUN 3

my baby in a[n] _____ and _____ outfit. The perfect way to
                     ADJECTIVE 4   COLOR 1

_____ all over town showing off my baby.
   VERB 2

Coming Out of BABY

Fill in the circles with the first words that come to mind when you hear the word "baby." Think about how you feel, the things you think about, what makes you happy or excited. There are no right or wrong answers!

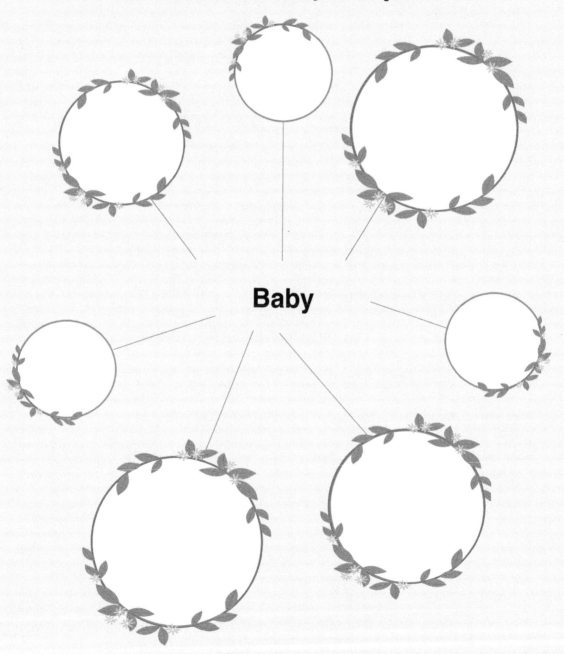

Baby

Serene Mama

Think of all the colors that bring you calmness right now, and use them as your color palette for this sweet mama.

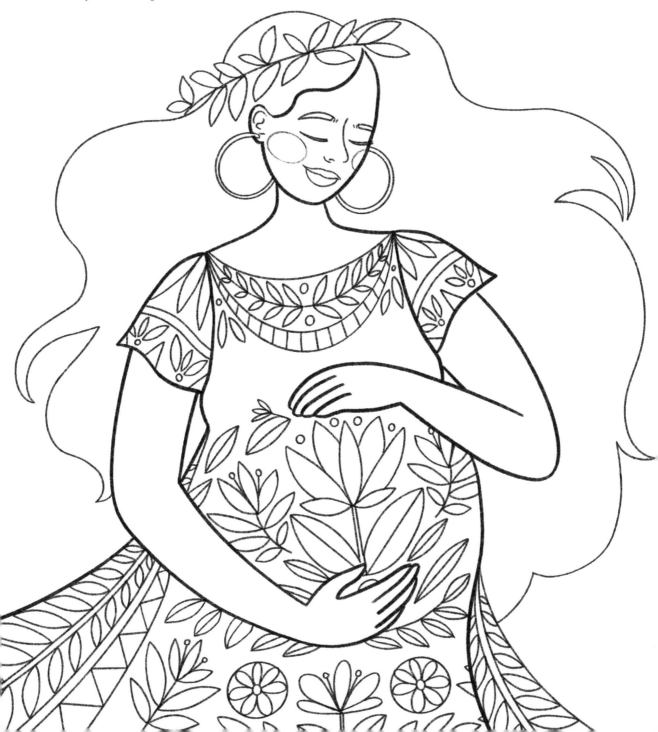

INFLUX OF EMOTIONS

Have you experienced a flow of tears while watching a commercial yet? Have you hurtled from joy over your growing belly straight into fear of what's to come?

As with any type of change, it's completely normal to feel and experience a range of emotions. Right now, your hormones are in overdrive. You've got the perfect recipe for heightened emotions and mood swings.

But you're not alone, and there are ways to cope with those unpredictable pregnancy emotions:

Sleep. While this may sound more like a fairy tale when you're expecting, there are ways to improve sleep. Eight hours should be the goal. Try different sleeping positions or purchase a body pillow to help. Chat with your partner about the sleep you need and, together, work out ways to help you get the rest you need. When your mind and body are restored, you can better handle the emotions as they come.

Healthy foods. Obviously a healthy diet is good for our physical body, but it's also good for our emotional well-being. Consuming less sugar and getting in those omega-3s and antioxidants can be a great way to help improve moods and balance emotions.

Self-care. When your body is going through the work and effort of building a human, it's especially important to set aside time to take care of yourself. If you're craving a bubble bath, longing to read a book, or dreaming of a massage or pedicure, go for it! While you're at it, let go of the guilt of taking time for yourself. Your body is doing plenty of hard work. Taking time to recharge is not only a good idea, it's a necessity.

Support system. Pregnancy is such a beautiful time, and to help you through these changing emotions, it's important to surround yourself with people who support you. Having a partner, family member, or close friend to talk to is essential when you're struggling.

Second Trimester Check-In

Fill in the prompts with the first words that come to mind. It's always fun to look back to see how you were feeling in these moments (ups and downs included!).

I am feeling _____

I am craving _____

I am thinking about _____

I have been eating _____

I can't stop watching _____

I am listening to _____

I am dreaming about _____

My favorite thing to do is _____

In the middle of the night I _____

I am laughing at _____

I have been wearing _____

What surprised me the most is _____

I'm most excited for _____

BUMP AWARENESS

Now that you're in the second trimester, you're likely noticing changes in your body other than just pains and nausea (which have hopefully subsided now!). With a growing belly, this trimester can be one of the most exciting. Usually you get a burst of energy, you start to lose the morning sickness, and your bump starts to show!

Unfortunately, as your baby is growing and your body is changing, some positions become uncomfortable. Your regular sleep positions might not work for you any longer.

Lying face down will start to be unpleasant, and sleeping on your back puts the weight of the abdomen on major blood vessels, intestines, back muscles, and spine. That pressure can lead to all kinds of issues, like hemorrhoids, backaches, and a decrease in blood circulation to you and your baby. As a result, your best sleep position is on your side with your knees bent. In fact, the American Pregnancy Association calls it SOS (sleep on side) and recommends your left side since that will increase circulation and the amount of nutrients that reach your baby.

If you're used to sleeping on your stomach or on your back, you should invest in a body pillow or use an extra pillow tucked between your legs for SOS. Fair warning here, don't freak out if you wake up to find you've moved into another position: You and your baby will be just fine! Try to get used to this new sleep position. In the long run, it will be the most comfortable one you can find.

As for sitting positions, as long as you're feeling comfortable and supported, you don't need to worry about a particular position. If you know you're going to be sitting for long periods of time, make sure to take short walk breaks to help with circulation. It might be more comfortable to add a small pillow behind your back. If you start to experience swelling, elevate your feet and increase the number of breaks to change positions frequently.

Mama in Repose

You'll hear it over and over: Rest while you can!
A woman at rest is a woman at her best.

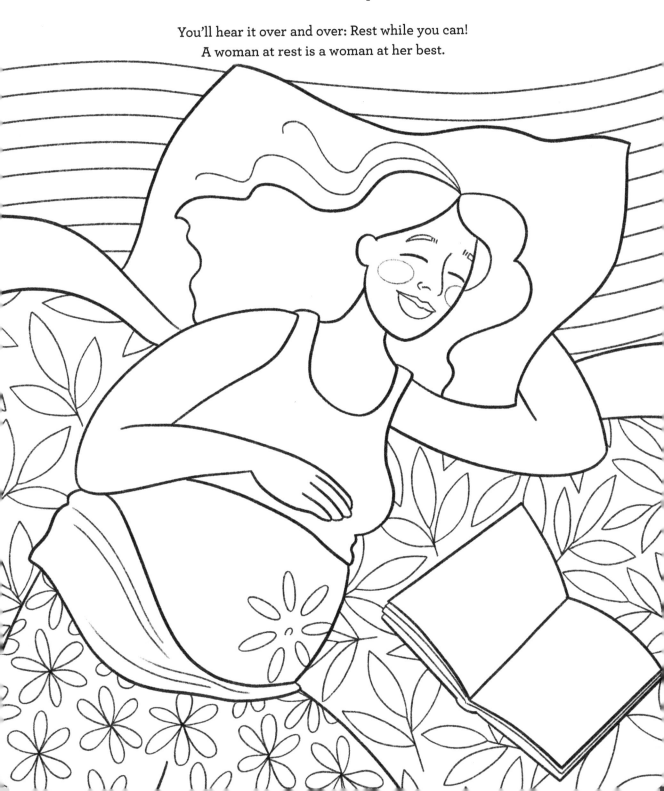

Name That Baby!

Ready to start thinking about baby names? This word association game will help you dream up creative names, and you can also use this as inspiration for your nursery decor, maternity shoot, and more! Without thinking too hard, fill in the blanks.

What name comes to mind when you think of your favorite song? _____

_____

What is your favorite city to visit? _____

What place is on your bucket list for a vacation? _____

What is your happy color? _____

What is your favorite color? _____

What city did you grow up in? _____

What is your favorite fruit? _____

Do you have relatives you'd like to name your baby after? _____

_____

Do you have a favorite family name? _____

What brings you joy? _____

_____

Do you have a favorite month? _____

What is your favorite season? _____

Do you have a favorite animated character? _____

Who was your childhood hero? _____

What is your birthstone? _____

What is the birthstone of the month with your baby's due date? _____

_____

Do you have a song you play when you are feeling loved? _____

_____

List the first three words that come to mind when you imagine meeting your

baby: _____

Look up synonyms in the thesaurus for those words and write your favorites

here: _____

_____

Did you find any name options that might be in the running? List them here: ____

_____

_____

Tip: Do an online search for the meanings behind the top names on your list.
Have fun with it, and don't worry. You can always make your final choices after
you're holding your sweet baby in your arms.

Pregnancy Needs

In your second trimester, you'll keep using lots of the same items from your first trimester, but you'll have new supplies and experiences, too. Complete the crossword by filling in a word or words that best fits each clue.

Across

2. How you want to deliver your baby
3. Clothing item that undergirds your bosom
4. Hands-on approach to relaxing the muscles
5. Specially formulated pill for you and baby
8. Learning what to do after your baby is born
10. Soft, comforting sleep buddy

Down

1. Up-close look at baby
4. Name for specially made attire when pregnant
5. Strengthening areas that help you with delivery
6. H_2O
7. Something to do on your side
9. Helps your body produce and maintain new cells
10. Questions for fluid in your veins
11. Supplies nourishment to dry areas on the body

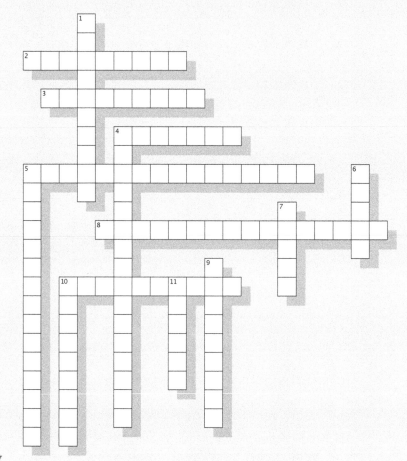

GESTATIONAL DIABETES

Let's face it, any testing that occurs during pregnancy can be nerve-racking . . . it's the fear of the unknown. But try not to panic when your doctor orders a new test. Many of them, like the glucose test, are a standard procedure for ALL pregnancies. Your doctor wants to uncover any possible complications so that they can do their best to treat you early on.

Your medical provider will usually test you for diabetes during a pregnancy. Of course, if you already have type 1 or 2 diabetes, make sure your doctor knows.

Most women who are not diabetic before pregnancy will be asked to take a glucose test between 26 and 28 weeks for what is known as gestational diabetes. Almost all women will be tested, regardless of their risk factors. The medical community has agreed that this glucose testing is the best way to catch signs of gestational diabetes. The test itself is mainly a blood draw to evaluate how your body processes sugar.

What to expect with a glucose screening test

- Fasting is not required. When you arrive for your test, they will have you drink a sweet liquid and then wait for one hour.
- After the hour, your blood is drawn. You won't know your results right away, but if the test is positive (meaning your body isn't processing the sugar correctly), your doctor will contact you for a follow-up test. Note that not everyone with a positive glucose screening has gestational diabetes.
- If a second test is needed and you're diagnosed, your doctor will most likely schedule you for more frequent visits and discuss a treatment plan. The doctor will need to make sure your body is producing enough insulin for you and your baby. Treating diabetes during pregnancy is important for you and the baby's health, which is why your doctor will be keeping a closer eye on you through routine testing.
- Only about 2 to 5 percent of women will get gestational diabetes, and it usually ends with the pregnancy. So relax, take a breath, and go with the flow. Always remember to ask your doctor if you're worried about something or have any questions.

Pregnancy Dreams

So many exciting and important things are happening while you're pregnant, but you can savor the smaller, more personal moments, too. Since pregnancy is likely to be a season of vivid dreams, take some time to reflect on them.

Describe your dream: _____

_____

_____

_____

_____

_____

_____

Draw a character or place from your dream:	Draw an image that conveys the main emotion of your dream:	Draw an image that existed only in the confines of your dream:

THE SCIENCE BEHIND PREGNANCY DREAMS

If you're having more intense dreams lately and you think the pregnancy might have something to do with it, you're right!

Remember those increased hormones that brought along SO many changes to your body and emotions in the first trimester? They aren't done with you yet.

Many women find that during pregnancy, they have much more vivid dreams that are easier to recall. Hormones likely play a part.

Your changing sleep cycles during pregnancy also play a role. A more tired body means deeper sleep, but at the same time, pregnant women tend to wake up frequently, often because they need to pee or move into a more comfortable position. Waking during REM (which is when dreams typically occur) means there's better dream recall, and the dreams feel more real and vivid.

The things we most often think about tend to show up in dreams, and during pregnancy, we women are thinking about pregnancy and childbirth pretty often (aka ALL THE TIME). Pregnancy, birth, and motherhood themes might show up in your hormone-induced vivid dreams.

Even bad dreams can be beneficial. In fact, The National Sleep Foundation claims that women who have nightmares about long, intense labors go on to have shorter and easier deliveries. So, don't be afraid of those dreams!

During your pregnancy, try jotting down your dreams in a journal. Recording what you're dreaming about can help you connect with your emotions, work through them, or even solve a problem. And if you're worried about sleep, try drinking less fluids right before bed and practice a relaxing evening routine. More colorful dreams are normal during pregnancy, and maybe it will be one of the things you enjoy about it!

Strike a Pose!

Capturing your pregnancy will mean a lot down the road. To help spark some ideas for your photo shoot, circle the words in this list that make you smile, and then fill in the blanks next to the prompts.

farm	outside	inside	beach
studio	professional	snow	sand
dress	pants	overalls	full makeup
all-natural	cityscape	running	walking
sitting	lifestyle	posed	coffee
alone	numbers	name	chalkboard
balloons	confetti	year	number 1
belly showing	park	travel	cozy
warm	fireplace	at home	baby room theme
significant location	friends	family	ultrasound
fields	flowers	trees	bridges
fancy	rugged	chic	barefoot

Fill in the blanks:

A place that has a special meaning to me is _____

A color that I associate with this pregnancy is _____

A special item that already means a lot to me is _____

Is there a theme or a main idea apparent? Are there any locations that would hold significance for you and this pregnancy?

_____

_____

Registry Necessities Scramble

It's never too early to start your baby registry, and since you don't have to share it with anyone right away, there's no time like the present. Unscramble the words to kick-start your baby registry!

aybb ttbelos _____

aficperi _____

piwes _____

seinoes _____

bsarte mpup _____

bbsi _____

ydob wolipl _____

byba tniomro _____

daprie gab _____

eslorltr _____

rac eats _____

hghi hacir _____

reidpas _____

plpnei raecm _____

beltot uhrsb _____

pubr shlotc _____

bcir _____

rcbi artssetm _____

dsleswad _____

kstaenlb _____

SELECTING YOUR SUPPORT TEAM

Good support goes a long way in helping you cope with both the physical and emotional changes that come in pregnancy as well as in labor. While it's good if you have a partner as a main source of support throughout your pregnancy and labor, one person can't do everything, which is why creating your own support team is essential. You may talk to some people on your team only a few times, while others can be there with you through most of your pregnancy. Nonetheless, all these people can and should support you in different ways.

What are some of the things a support team can help you with?

- Help you relax.
- Listen to you vent.
- Attend prenatal appointments and classes with you.
- Share a healthy lifestyle with you, including physical activities and meal preparation both during and after pregnancy.
- Help prepare your home for the baby's arrival.
- Read books with you.
- Share ideas and talk through plans for parenting.
- Take over household chores that aren't safe for you, like helping you with chemical cleaning products, lifting heavy items, and cleaning your cat's litter box.
- Talk through a birth plan with you.
- Help with assembling baby gear.

You're a powerful woman, and your body is doing something amazing right now. Also, there are things that you can't physically do. Having a team of people who support you can help the entire process be a positive experience.

Your professional support team will help answer questions that may arise related to the physical side of your pregnancy. This healthcare team will include individuals such as your doctor or midwife, dentist, and/or OB-GYN. If your pregnancy is high-risk, like pregnancies with twins, you might have a fetal doctor called a perinatologist. You might want further support from a lactation consultant, a doula, a chiropractor, or a naturopath.

For your personal support team, enlist your partner, friends, and family that you feel close to. You may also want to lean on other expecting mothers from prenatal classes.

Having a group of people who lift you up is a great way to set yourself up for an easier pregnancy.

Boy, Girl, or Big Surprise?

If you haven't decided whether you want to find out the gender of your baby, these prompts will help you choose! Answer each of the questions or finish the sentence with what first comes to mind.

Pros of waiting until birth:

I want to be surprised because _____

I've long been a fan of the unexpected, like _____

The sex of my baby is one of life's greatest surprises, and I don't want to _____

_____

All that matters is having a healthy _____

If I know my baby's gender, I might start to develop _____

I'll avoid receiving too many gender-specific _____ and toys.

I want to have a surprise to look forward to at the end of _____

Pros of knowing before birth:

I've always wanted to have a reveal party and invite _____

I'm a planner and want to use _____ as a color theme.

I want to develop a bond, and knowing the gender would help this baby feel more

_____

I've had my mind set on having a _____

and would like the time to make peace with whatever my doctor tells me.

I have plans for _____

as the name and need to know if I need to come up with another one.

Friends and family will have an easier time buying _____

_____

Pregnancy Aches and Pains

In a dream world, pregnancy would be all about that dewy glow and that cute belly. But this is the real world, so complete this crossword about some of the less pleasant side effects of bringing life into this world.

Across

1. Hard to move from one place to another
4. Enlarged area between leg and foot
5. Hurting cabeza (Spanish)
11. Unable to stop moving legs
12. Rudolph the red _____ reindeer + what happens when you get cut
13. Not high and periodic table Mg
14. Fake news when it comes to contractions

Down

2. Muscle that didn't sign up for this movement
3. Chewing _____ + another word for tenderness
6. Sore synonym + rhymes with Elvis
7. More than a _____ + another word for woozy
8. What holds your uterus to your lower back
9. Tightness at the end of spine
10. Another way to say charley horse

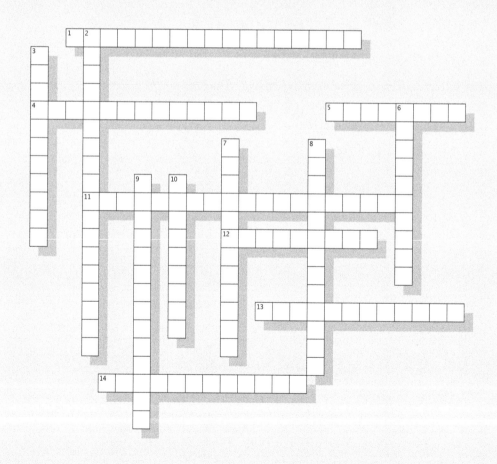

WHAT IS PREECLAMPSIA?

It's not fun to talk about some of the complications that can arise during pregnancy, but it's helpful to be prepared, just in case. And your doctor will know just what to do. Preeclampsia is a complication of pregnancy that can cause high blood pressure, kidney damage, and other serious issues for mothers and babies. It affects about 5 to 8 percent of all pregnancies. Preeclampsia usually begins after 20 weeks, but it can develop at any time during a pregnancy, during labor, and for up to six weeks after delivery. Preeclampsia can develop even if you feel fine—and it can progress slowly or quickly. This is one of the reasons your doctor tests your urine throughout your pregnancy: They're looking for protein levels that indicate the onset of preeclampsia.

The symptoms of preeclampsia vary from woman to woman and aren't always noticeable, especially when you don't know what to look for and are in the early stages of the condition. Symptoms include sudden swelling in the hands and face (especially around the eyes), changes in vision that include blurry vision, temporary loss of vision, or light sensitivity, severe headaches, and shortness of breath. You'll notice that some of these symptoms are similar to typical pregnancy complications, so they may go unnoticed. It's also worth noting that not every woman who has swelling has preeclampsia.

While it can sound scary, and while preeclampsia is a condition to be taken seriously, talk to your doctor about it, especially if you notice swelling! If you're at risk, your doctor might suggest starting an aspirin regimen prior to 16 weeks gestation.

Bumped into New Symptoms

As your belly is getting bigger, strangers might notice you're pregnant, and you might notice some strange new symptoms. Unscramble these words and see if you can relate.

lge carpsm   — — — — — — — — —

gegbir leybl   — — — — — — — — — — —

gesoclu estt   — — — — — — — — — —

kacechbac   — — — — — — — — —

terwa ereteoint   — — — — — — — — — — — — —

sidizisinze   — — — — — — — — — —

cslmue spsmas   — — — — — — — — — — — —

deicrsaen odod scrngvai   — — — — — — — — — — — —

— — — — — — — — —

idviv meadsr   — — — — — — — — — —

rnraebunhtr   — — — — — — — — — —

degleinb gsum   — — — — — — — — — —

waledd kwla   — — — — — — — — — —

sthcloe ton gttfini   — — — — — — — — — — — —

— — — — —

nedert sreatbs   — — — — — — — — — — — — —

nlaie agrne   — — — — — — — — — —

SECOND TRIMESTER SYMPTOMS

Symptoms can be scary at first, especially as a first-time mom. Remember, your body knows what to do. Yes, you may be feeling different from how you used to, but that is completely normal. Sometimes, symptoms can linger or become a little more than what you're comfortable with. This is where a good relationship with your doctor is a powerful tool to ease your mind.

Even though the second trimester is usually one of the most enjoyable, here are a few other symptoms that may make an appearance in the second trimester and some ways to ease them.

Round Ligament Pain

You may ocassionally feel sharp or shooting pains in your lower back when walking or exercising. This is common as you enter the second trimester and is referred to as "round ligament pain." In a nutshell, there are two ligaments that hold up the uterus as it grows. The bigger your belly gets, the harder they have to work to hold the uterus up. Many women have found relief in stretching or prenatal yoga classes. As always, check with your OB-GYN before undertaking any new exercise.

Growing Belly and Breasts

It's no secret that your belly grows along with your growing baby, especially in the second and third trimesters. But along with an expanding abdomen, your breasts will also consistently increase in size. A good supportive bra as well as supportive belly bands can help with your discomfort.

Skin Changes

Your hormone changes and your growing body will probably trigger changes in your skin as well. Pregnancy often increases the pigment in your skin called melanin. You might see brown patches on your face, called melasma, and a dark line that runs down from your belly button, called a linea nigra. Both of these skin changes are harmless and usually fade after pregnancy, but they can be darkened or aggravated by sun exposure, so be sure to wear sunscreen outdoors.

Nasal Changes

As your body makes more blood during pregnancy, mucus membranes may start to swell and give you a stuffy nose. Drinking plenty of fluids, using a humidifier, and using a saline rinse can all help relieve congestion.

Leg Cramps

Waking up in the middle of the night with a pregnancy leg cramp is common, even though it's not something often talked about. While it's not certain what causes the leg cramps specifically, there are a few ways to reduce or prevent them. Drink plenty of fluids, avoid sitting or standing in one position for extended periods, and stretch before bed. You can also take a warm bath or shower before bed to relax the leg muscles. If a cramp does occur, try a warm compress or gentle stretching.

Dizziness

Due to changes in your hormones and blood circulation, pregnancy can leave you feeling dizzy. If this is something you're experiencing, drink plenty of fluids (hydration helps!) and move slowly to make sure you've regained your balance when standing or sitting. Avoid standing in the same position for long periods. Eating regularly will also help ward off large dips in blood sugar levels. If you still feel faint, lie down on your side.

Urinary Tract Infection

UTIs are actually very common during pregnancy because of the added pressure a fetus can place on the bladder and urinary tract. Sometimes UTIs can be detected from your standard urine tests before you even feel any symptoms. Of course, if you do feel pain when urinating or if you have a fever, reach out to your doctor right away. A UTI is easily treatable with antibiotics, and you don't want to let it linger.

Dental Issues

Pregnancy itself doesn't immediately affect your teeth, but the change in hormones may cause your teeth or gums to become more sensitive; it also increases your risk of gum disease. Frequent vomiting can also affect your tooth enamel, so it's important to take care of your teeth while you're pregnant. Keep up with your regular dental appointments and let your dentist know that you're expecting so they can examine your gums.

Second Trimester Checklist

For many women, this is the easiest of the three trimesters of pregnancy, so it's the perfect time to take advantage of that burst of energy by preparing for your baby's arrival. If you're wondering what you can do to prepare right now, since that due date still feels so far away, we've rounded up plenty to keep you busy with that second trimester energy!

☐ Decide on your pregnancy announcement and share the news with friends and family.

☐ Schedule your 20-week ultrasound. This is the time you can find out the gender of your baby, so decide ahead of time and remind the nursing staff, technicians, and doctor if you want to be surprised—you don't want them to let it slip.

☐ Create your baby registry.

☐ Start sleeping on your side.

☐ Ask for recommendations from friends and family to help find a pediatrician who aligns with your preferences and parenting philosophy.

☐ Get your teeth cleaned. Pregnancy increases the risk of gum disease, so getting a cleaning is not only safe but recommended.

☐ Start thinking about your baby shower and decide on details like the host, the location, the budget, and the date. Typically, you'll have your shower between 24 and 32 weeks.

☐ Enroll in childbirth or baby care classes at your hospital.

☐ Ask your doctor about scheduling your glucose screening test for 24 to 28 weeks.

☐ If you're going to need childcare, start your childcare search and schedule tours with your top choices.

☐ Decide if you're going to hire a doula to be your professional labor coach.

☐ Consider going on a "babymoon"—one last vacation with only you and your partner before the baby comes.

Getting through the Hump

Pregnancy comes with plenty of twists and turns. Help this mama navigate her way to holding her beautiful baby bump.

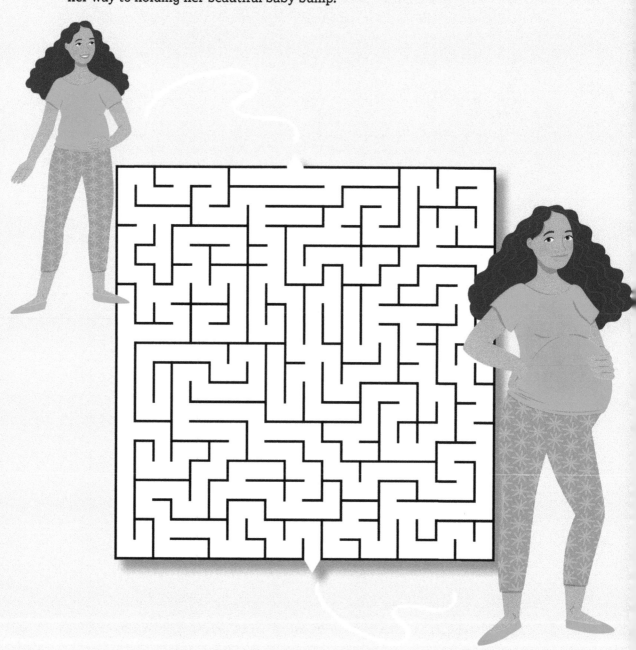

Dear Baby

This letter can be such a beautiful memento to share with your little one later. It doesn't have to be perfect; just let the words come from your heart. Consider writing about what things you are most looking forward to doing with your baby, or what being a mother means to you.

_____

_____

_____

_____

_____

_____

_____

_____

_____

_____

_____

_____

_____

_____

_____

Pregnancy Dos and Don'ts

Using the lists, find and circle the dos and don'ts during pregnancy. Look for them in all directions, including backward and diagonally..

Dos

Hydrate	Journal	Belly photos
Walks	Ultrasound	Massage
Rest	Vitamins	Dentist
Moisturize	Swim	Registry

Don'ts

Raw meat	Smoke	X-ray
Paint	Sauna	Scuba dive
Stilettos	Cat litter	
Hot tub	Alcohol	

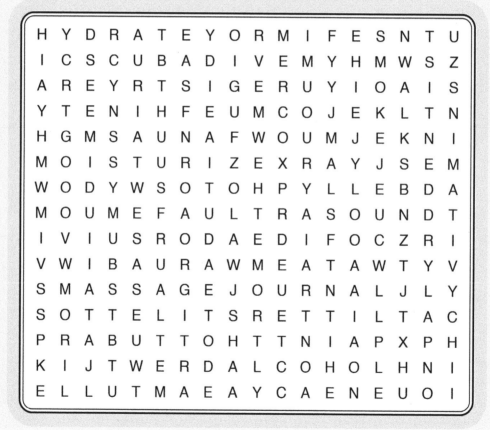

H Y D R A T E Y O R M I F E S N T U
I C S C U B A D I V E M Y H M W S Z
A R E Y R T S I G E R U Y I O A I S
Y T E N I H F E U M C O J E K L T N
H G M S A U N A F W O U M J E K N I
M O I S T U R I Z E X R A Y J S E M
W O D Y W S O T O H P Y L L E B D A
M O U M E F A U L T R A S O U N D T
I V I U S R O D A E D I F O C Z R I
V W I B A U R A W M E A T A W T Y V
S M A S S A G E J O U R N A L J L Y
S O T T E L I T S R E T T I L T A C
P R A B U T T O H T T N I A P X P H
K I J T W E R D A L C O H O L H N I
E L L U T M A E A Y C A E N E U O I

EXPECTING SEX

Now that you've conceived, is it still safe to do the deed? Just about every expecting mama (and probably her partner) has this question on her mind.

Most doctors and OB-GYNs agree that during any normal, healthy pregnancy, sex is completely safe and even encouraged. Since there is so much focus on the baby and your changing body for those nine months, it's easy for your romantic relationship to fall by the wayside. Intimacy is important for feeling close to your partner, as long as you're feeling up for it.

The second trimester is sometimes even referred to as the "honeymoon phase" because much of the nauseating first trimester symptoms have passed, your belly and breasts have grown to a comfortable size, and an increase in blood flow can heighten sensitivity throughout all your erogenous zones. Typically, the added energy and hormones of the second trimester also mean an increase in libido.

What it comes down to is this: Don't be afraid of intimacy during pregnancy. Pregnancy can be life-altering enough, and sex is something that you don't have to stop because of it. If you're worried about the safety of your baby, you're not alone. Rest assured, though, your baby is well cocooned in amniotic fluid, safely away from the vagina, behind the cervix, and within the walls of the uterus.

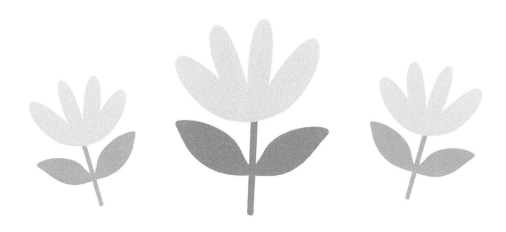

What's in a Pregnancy?

How many three letter words can you make using the letters in PREGNANCY?

_____   _____

_____   _____

_____   _____

_____   _____

_____   _____

_____   _____

_____   _____

_____   _____

_____   _____

_____   _____

_____   _____

_____   _____

_____   _____

_____   _____

_____   _____

_____   _____

Preeclampsia

Make sure to familiarize yourself with the symptoms of preeclampsia (page 53).
Then answer True or False to the following questions.

It's a possible sign of preeclampsia if:

1. You have a severe headache that won't subside with over-the-counter drugs like acetaminophen. T / F

2. You have blurry or double vision, vision loss, or light sensitivity. T / F

3. A doctor says you have certain protein in your urine. T / F

4. Your belly is growing. T / F

5. You are experiencing excessive weight gain not related to eating. T / F

6. You are out of breath often when doing light activities. T / F

7. You have a lot of sudden swelling in the hands and face. T / F

8. Your stomach hurts, especially in the upper abdomen area. T / F

9. You are having heartburn quite frequently after eating. T / F

10. You are peeing less, and when you urinate, the urine is dark and smelly. T / F

11. Your ankles have been swollen for a long time and it feels like a constant muscle cramp. T / F

12. You smile a lot thinking of your baby. T / F

13. You want to eat junk foods. T / F

14. Your blood pressure is above normal and that's not like you. T / F

First Time I . . .

Fill in the blanks to document the first time you feel your baby move. Babies start to move much earlier than this, but sometime between week 16 and week 25 is when you can feel these movements.

The first time I felt baby move I was...

thinking _____

wearing _____

listening to _____

eating _____

going _____

dreaming of _____

feeling _____

had to tell _____

Pregnancy Milestones!

Fill in the date or write down a memory of each of these milestones.

Positive pregnancy test ⎯⎯⎯⎯⎯⎯⎯⎯⎯⎯⎯⎯⎯⎯⎯⎯⎯⎯

First time I told someone ⎯⎯⎯⎯⎯⎯⎯⎯⎯⎯⎯⎯⎯⎯⎯⎯⎯

First doctor appointment ⎯⎯⎯⎯⎯⎯⎯⎯⎯⎯⎯⎯⎯⎯⎯⎯⎯

First time hearing heartbeat ⎯⎯⎯⎯⎯⎯⎯⎯⎯⎯⎯⎯⎯⎯⎯

First craving ⎯⎯⎯⎯⎯⎯⎯⎯⎯⎯⎯⎯⎯⎯⎯⎯⎯⎯⎯⎯⎯⎯⎯

First ultrasound ⎯⎯⎯⎯⎯⎯⎯⎯⎯⎯⎯⎯⎯⎯⎯⎯⎯⎯⎯⎯⎯

First time feeling the baby kick ⎯⎯⎯⎯⎯⎯⎯⎯⎯⎯⎯⎯⎯

First time feeling hiccups ⎯⎯⎯⎯⎯⎯⎯⎯⎯⎯⎯⎯⎯⎯⎯⎯

First time wearing maternity clothing ⎯⎯⎯⎯⎯⎯⎯⎯⎯

Day you found out gender ⎯⎯⎯⎯⎯⎯⎯⎯⎯⎯⎯⎯⎯⎯⎯⎯

First baby outfit purchased ⎯⎯⎯⎯⎯⎯⎯⎯⎯⎯⎯⎯⎯⎯⎯

First time you noticed a real baby bump ⎯⎯⎯⎯⎯⎯⎯⎯

First time someone else felt the baby kick ⎯⎯⎯⎯⎯⎯⎯

First baby gift ⎯⎯⎯⎯⎯⎯⎯⎯⎯⎯⎯⎯⎯⎯⎯⎯⎯⎯⎯⎯⎯⎯

First sign of labor ⎯⎯⎯⎯⎯⎯⎯⎯⎯⎯⎯⎯⎯⎯⎯⎯⎯⎯⎯⎯

A Fearsome Craving

Write down the first word that first comes to mind when you read the following parts of speech. Then read the story aloud using the words from your list. Try reading this aloud with a partner.

NOUN 1 _____

VERB 1 (ending in -ed) _____

NOUN 2 _____

NOUN 3 _____

VERB 2 (ending in -ing) _____

COLOR _____

ADJECTIVE _____

ADJECTIVE 2 _____

NOUN 4 _____

VERB 3 (ending in -ed) _____

ADJECTIVE 3 _____

ANIMAL _____

ADJECTIVE 4 _____

I woke up in the middle of the night and just had a craving for _____ . So
NOUN 1

I _____ out of bed and grabbed my _____ before I made my
VERB 1 (ending in -ed)   NOUN 2

way to the driveway to get into my _____.
NOUN 3

I drove so fast it was like I was _____. The only place open was
VERB 2 (ending in -ing)

this _____ _____ greasy spoon. As I walked through the creaky door,
COLOR ADJECTIVE

I caught a glimpse of myself in the mirror and couldn't believe how _____
ADJECTIVE 2

my hair was. Before I knew it, my hand was rifling through my bag for a _____
NOUN 4

for a quick-fix. Once I _____ my hair, I couldn't help but order a
VERB 3 (ending in -ed)

heaping serving of _____. This baby was like a _____ trying to
NOUN 1   ADJECTIVE 3 (ANIMAL)

claw for food.

After I gorged myself on _____, I sat in the booth with a _____ smile on
NOUN 1   ADJECTIVE 4

my face. I was satisfied. Until the next craving.

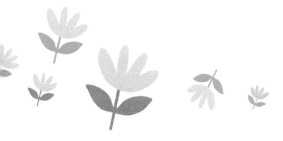

What's Going On in There?

How much do you know about your little one? Test your knowledge with this quiz and see if you can figure out the crazy amount of changes as your baby grows.

1. **At the beginning of the second trimester, what is the biggest part of the baby?**
    A. Feet

    B. Hands

    C. Stomach

    D. Head

2. **Choose the one that happens during the second trimester:**
    A. The baby's heart starts beating.

    B. The baby can begin to see.

    C. The baby can start to frown.

    D. The baby starts to recognize words.

3. **How long will your baby be by the end of the second trimester?**
    A. 4 inches

    B. 9 inches

    C. 7 inches

    D. 12 inches

4. **What will your baby have by end of second trimester?**
    A. Name and Social Security card

    B. Fingerprints and footprints

    C. A full head of hair

    D. Ambition

5. **What does the phrase "from crown to rump" mean?**
    A. The baby's length from the top of its head to its butt.

    B. My tooth is falling out.

    C. The fall of a king.

    D. The bean-like shape of a 13-week-old fetus.

6. **What bodily function will baby begin to do during the second trimester?**
    A. Sneeze

    B. Cough

    C. Urinate

    D. Defecate

7. **My doctor should be able to identify the sex of the baby during this trimester.**

   T / F

8. **What sensation do most women have in their bellies when they start to notice their baby moving?**
   A. Motion sickness
   B. Stomach dropping
   C. Sharp pain
   D. Fluttering or bubbling

9. **At around week 17, what does the baby start developing?**
   A. Mucus
   B. Blood
   C. Umbilical cord
   D. Toenails

10. **A baby develops a thin, shiny coating on its skin during the second trimester. What is it called?**
    A. Trailmix
    B. Larnyx
    C. Vernix
    D. Coatex

11. **At the end of the fifth month, the baby is about _____ inches long.**
    A. 12
    B. 6
    C. 4
    D. 9

12. **During second trimester the baby's first poop appears in its intestines. What is it called?**
    A. Meconium
    B. Magnesium
    C. Plutonium
    D. Sodium

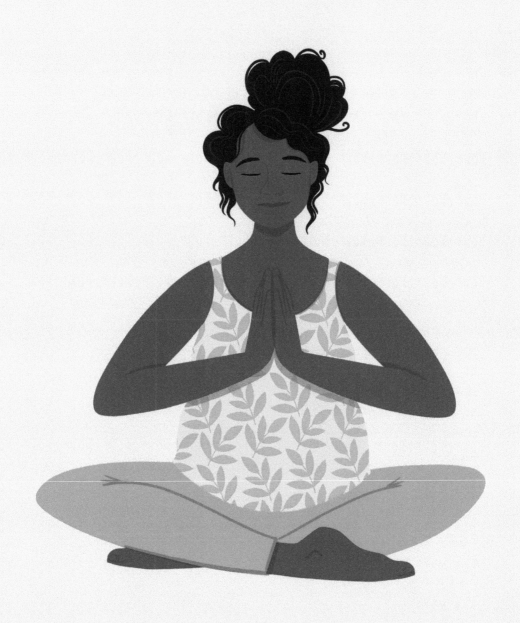

Third Trimester

(28 TO 40 WEEKS)

Third Trimester Expectations Checklist

Check off the list as you experience each week!

☐ 28 Weeks: Checkups will probably be scheduled every two weeks between now and week 32, depending on your pregnancy and your doctor.

☐ 29 Weeks: It's not uncommon for blood pressure to rise a little. If you experience severe headaches, blurred vision, or sudden swelling around the face, let your doctor know.

☐ 30 Weeks: Around this week of pregnancy, your baby weighs around 3 pounds and probably has hair.

☐ 31 Weeks: At this point, your baby will start rapidly gaining weight.

☐ 32 Weeks: Your baby's hearing is getting more sensitive. Keep talking and singing to your baby.

☐ 33 Weeks: Your baby's bones are starting to harden, although the skull will remain flexible.

☐ 34 Weeks: Your baby has a full set of fingernails by now.

☐ 35 Weeks: Your doctor will schedule a Group B Streptococcus screening between 35 and 37 weeks to detect if you need antibiotics during delivery to protect the baby.

☐ 36 Weeks: You start having weekly checkups.

☐ 37 Weeks: If you haven't already, this is a good time to think about whether you want to breastfeed. It can be helpful to consult a lactation expert.

☐ 38 Weeks: Your breasts are now producing colostrum—the special nutrient-rich milk that will nourish your baby in the first days. Don't be surprised by a little wetness or yellow marks in your bra.

☐ 39 Weeks: Your baby is considered full term.

☐ 40 Weeks: You're almost there! Birth could happen at any time (and up to 2 weeks later than your due date). Don't be alarmed if you don't deliver right away.

HOSPITAL BAG PREP

Everyone is different, but overall, these are some items you'll probably be happy to have at the hospital. Is everything a necessity? No. You could show up with nothing in hand and be fine. But this is about making that hospital stay as comfortable as possible!

It's wise to pack a hospital bag between 32 and 35 weeks and have everything ready to go by week 35 in case you have an early delivery. No matter when you start packing, though, remember that for labor and delivery, you are priority number one. The doctors will focus on you and your baby, and there will special staff on hand to care for your baby. The focus of your hospital prep should be all about providing you with the items you may need to get you through labor and the time after delivery as comfortably as possible.

At the very least, you'll want a few essentials, but go ahead and skip the blow dryer and curling iron . . . nobody's got time for that! Typically, a ponytail or bun is where it's at. Make sure to have on hand what makes YOU feel the most like YOU. If it's a favorite shower gel, then pack it. If it's a certain lip color, stash it in your bag. You probably want to invest in travel-size versions of the essentials so they don't take up so much room in your bag and you can have them ready beforehand.

What to pack

You won't need to bring too much to the hospital for the birth, and if you have an uncomplicated vaginal delivery, you may be there for only a day or two. If you are going in for a planned C-section, you will likely recover in the hospital for two to four days after having this surgery, so you'll definitely want to keep that in mind when you're preparing.

- **Loose clothing that won't press on your incision.** Avoid pants, elastic on the waist, and zippers! Nursing nightgowns are perfect, and a flowy dress is a great idea for going back home.
- **A binder or wrap to support your belly.** The hospital may provide this, so it's good to ask ahead of time.
- **Prescription medication and prenatal vitamins**. Bring enough for four days.

What your partner should pack

Your partner could be your rock or could be a mess seeing you in pain. But a comfortable partner will be better able to focus on you. While your partner won't need to take a ton, there are some items your copilot might want to stash in the hospital go-bag.

- A change of clothes
- An extra pair of pajamas, underwear, and socks
- A casual shirt for in-hospital photos
- Toothbrush and deodorant
- Twin sheet set (optional)

What not to pack in your delivery bag

There are many things the hospital will provide to save you precious space in your delivery bag, so be sure to take advantage of these and don't be afraid to ask for extras! However, if you are at a birth center, check with them ahead of time to see what they have on hand, and be sure to ask about diapers and wipes.

- Diapers, wipes, onesies, a hat, a swaddle blanket (pack these items only if there's a specific color or brand you want)
- Tylenol and Tums
- Colace or another stool softener
- Dermoplast or other numbing spray
- Mesh panties and pads
- Tucks pads, ice pads, and other hemorrhoid treatments

Hospital Bag Checklist

Check off the following items as you prepare your hospital go-bag.

Checklist for Mama:

- ☐ Robe
- ☐ Slippers
- ☐ Nightgown
- ☐ Socks
- ☐ Shower sandals
- ☐ Nursing bra
- ☐ Nursing pads
- ☐ Nipple cream
- ☐ Going home outfit
- ☐ Lip balm
- ☐ Hair ties
- ☐ Toiletries

Checklist for Baby:

- ☐ Diaper bag
- ☐ Going home outfit
- ☐ Hat
- ☐ Pacifier
- ☐ Swaddle
- ☐ Car seat

Mama's Little Self-Helper

While your body is busy doing so much, but you have the time . . . it's the perfect opportunity to take some extra care of yourself. Fill in the word that best completes each clue to reveal recommendations for self-care.

Dog command + a plus sign = __ __ __ __

__ __ __ __ __ __ __ __

Most important meal of the day + in + a place to lay your head =

__ __ __ __ __ __ __ __ __ in __ __ __

An old discipline from India + what you do in front of a camera =

__ __ __ __ __ __ __ __ __

Opposite of vanilla + a place where adult beverages are served =

__ __ __ __ __ __ __ __ __ __ __

Antonym for cool + white liquid produced by a cow =

__ __ __ __ __ __ __ __

Use gum to blow this + warm water in a tub =

__ __ __ __ __ __ __ __ __ __

A small human + a natural satellite of a planet =

__ __ __ __ __ __ __

Electrical energy + cats love them =

__ __ __ __ __ __ __ __

Calming down after a long day + vocal or instrumental sounds =

__ __ __ __ __ __ __ __ __ __ __ __ __

A place to record thoughts and feelings + to be granted access to an event =

__ __ __ __ __ __ __ __ __ __ __

Put Yourself First

Although there's a ton of pressure to build your entire life around your new baby, you're still a person with your own needs, and you have to have a plan for addressing them. Without thinking too much through each answer, fill in the blanks with whatever comes to mind. Use some of your answers to work on self-care right now.

I feel better when I _____

I feel taken care of when I _____

I feel stronger when I _____

Ways I like to relax: _____

_____

_____

_____

_____

Ways I can stay active: _____

_____

_____

_____

_____

If I were to do something lovely for me, it would be: _____

_____

_____

_____

_____

TAKE A LOAD OFF

During the second trimester, your hormones begin to level off a little. Most women feel more energetic, which is partly why this is the easiest trimester for most moms.

As you enter into the third trimester, you'll begin to feel more fatigue. With the baby getting bigger every day, you'll be tired from carrying the extra weight in your uterus. Your body is putting a lot of energy into growing your baby. At the same time, your pregnancy can be so physically uncomfortable that it might be hard to get a good night's sleep.

You're definitely not alone in the struggle. According to The National Sleep Foundation, 78 percent of women sleep more poorly during their pregnancies. Between heartburn, getting up to pee, physical discomfort, and emotional challenges, a good night's sleep can start to seem like an impossible dream. But there is hope!

If you're having trouble getting in those 8 to 10 hours of sleep recommended for pregnant women, try some of these methods to help.

- Make an actual sleep plan, including naps if needed.
- Get in some physical activity for at least 30 minutes per day.
- Sleep on your left side with knees and hips bent to improve blood flow and nutrients to your growing baby and your organs. Try to avoid lying on your back for extended periods of time.
- Invest in a good body pillow, or place pillows between your knees, under your growing stomach, and behind your back to help relieve lower back pressure.
- While you need to be drinking plenty of water throughout the day, cut down your fluid intake a few hours before bedtime.
- Especially in the third trimester, you'll be getting up frequently to urinate, but turning on a bright bathroom light can make it harder to fall back to sleep quickly. Instead, place a nightlight in the bathroom.
- Heartburn often gets worse when you lie down. To combat heartburn, try eating frequent small meals during the day and avoid large amounts of spicy, acidic, or fried foods, especially in the evening.
- Create a soothing evening routine. Avoid electronics or screens before bedtime. Try taking a warm bath, reading a book, knitting something for your baby, or whatever else relaxes you.

Baby Shower Blitz

Quickly answer these prompts with the first word that comes to mind and see if it serves to help in planning the theme of your baby shower! Don't edit yourself; just speed through it.

FAVORITE color _____

FAVORITE food _____

FAVORITE animal _____

FAVORITE book _____

FAVORITE song _____

FAVORITE place _____

FAVORITE movie _____

FAVORITE character _____

FAVORITE phrase _____

FAVORITE person _____

FAVORITE hobby _____

FAVORITE city _____

FAVORITE dessert _____

FAVORITE thing that makes you laugh

_____

FAVORITE drink _____

FAVORITE thing about nature _____

_____

Now think about what you wrote down. How could some of these answers go together for the baby shower of your dreams?

_____

_____

_____

_____

_____

_____

10 Things Baby Doesn't Need

There's already a long list of items you'll need, especially for your first baby, but there are a few things you can totally avoid purchasing. To cut down on clutter, unscramble these words to see what you can cross off of your shopping list or nix from your registry.

bayb selowt __ __ __ __ __ __ __ __ __ __

bbay oreb __ __ __ __ __ __ __ __

epswi aerrmw __ __ __ __ __ __ __ __ __ __ __

bayb ilo __ __ __ __ __ __ __

ooigbe eispw __ __ __ __ __ __ __ __ __ __

aciifepr seiwp __ __ __ __ __ __ __ __ __ __ __ __

fdetusf amlanis __ __ __ __ __ __ __ __ __ __ __ __ __

eenbnowr osseh __ __ __ __ __ __ __ __ __ __ __ __

hbta rmttremehoe __ __ __ __ __ __ __ __ __ __ __ __ __ __

tetobl ramerw __ __ __ __ __ __ __ __ __ __ __ __

Get the Pregnant Woman
to the Bathroom

Expect to pee even more frequently during the third trimester as your baby's growth adds even more pressure on your bladder. Help this pregnant mama find the bathroom!

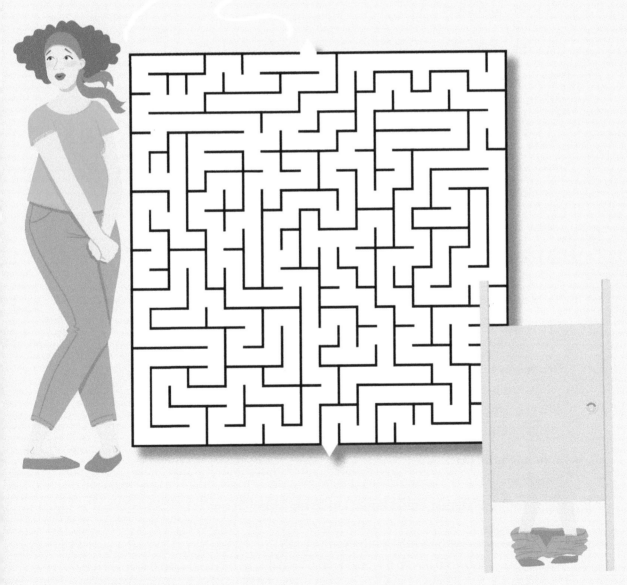

WEIRD PREGNANCY FACTS

Obviously your body is doing something amazing by growing a person. But your body is also going through its own sometimes bizarre physical changes. This is how a pregnancy might change you.

Your heart works harder.
Because your blood volume increases up to 60 percent during pregnancy, your heart has to pump 30 to 40 percent more blood per minute to keep it all flowing.

Your feet may grow.
Many women report their feet grow up to one size larger during pregnancy. Sometimes the change is permanent.

Yes, you probably will pee yourself.
There could be a few times you've wondered if your water broke. If you've got a continuous trickle or a sudden large gush, it most likely did. More often, though, pee just leaks out . . . one of those fun facts of pregnancy.

Your sense of smell can change during pregnancy.
Have you had those moments where you're asking everyone if they can smell that, too? It's a real phenomenon. Some say women's heightened sense of smell is to help protect them from unsafe foods.

Your hips widen.
Along with a growing abdomen, your pelvic bone actually separates in the middle. It's all caused by hormones, which will ultimately make it easier for you to give birth. The relaxing of joints is also part of the reason you tend to waddle toward the end of pregnancy.

Pregnancy brain is a real thing.
While it's not completely clear what causes the brain fog or trouble with memory at times, it happens. But with all the hormone changes, stress, and exhaustion of a pregnancy, it's no wonder we don't always think clearly.

Your boobs might leak.
It's not uncommon to lactate during pregnancy. Lactation may even be triggered by hearing another baby cry.

Mommy Hopes . . .

You haven't met your baby yet, but like every mom-to-be, you're dreaming of what they'll be like. Fill in the blanks as a fun memento to share with your child in the future. You'll see what came true—and just how much they've become their own person!

I hope you become _____

_____

I hope you love _____

_____

I hope you find _____

_____

I hope you learn _____

_____

I hope you laugh _____

_____

I hope you see _____

_____

I hope you always know _____

_____

I hope you remember _____

_____

When I heard you were on the way, I thought _____

_____

A special place I hope you visit someday is _____

_____

A Picture-Perfect Pregnancy

Have you scheduled your maternity photo shoot? Take a moment to imagine the colors and feel of your picture perfect maternity shoot!

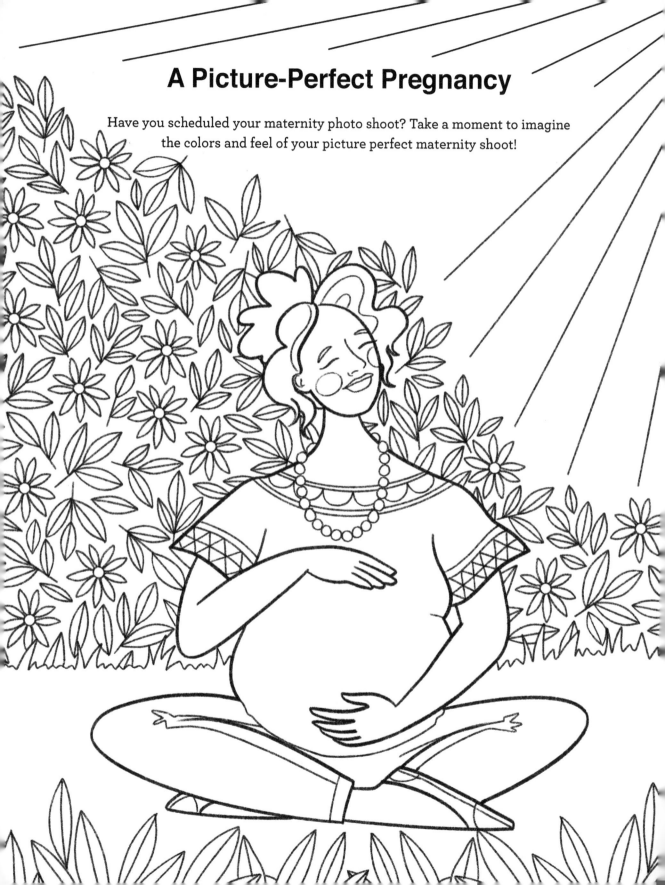

Baby's Family Tree

Start with your baby at the base of the tree and trace back as far as you'd like to go, both on your side and on your partner's. Add in any dates and locations you know, too.

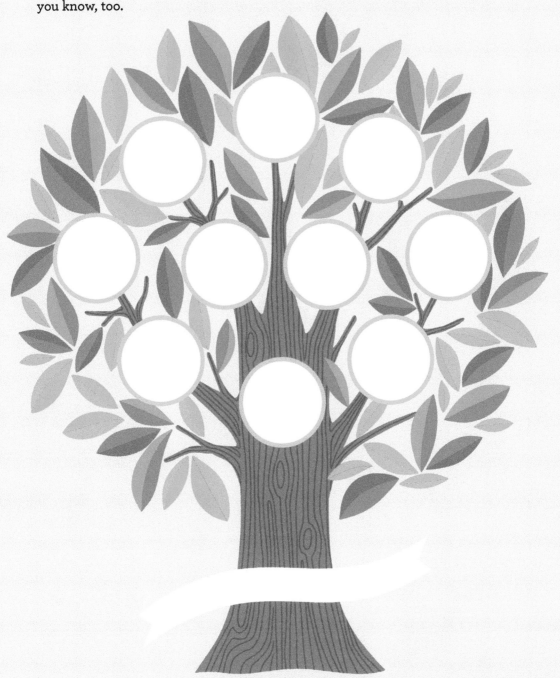

EXPECTING More Words

Look at the word EXPECTING. Then, at the end of each line radiating from EXPECTING, quickly write down the first word that comes to mind. Try not to pause or think too much. When you're finished, reflect on what you wrote.

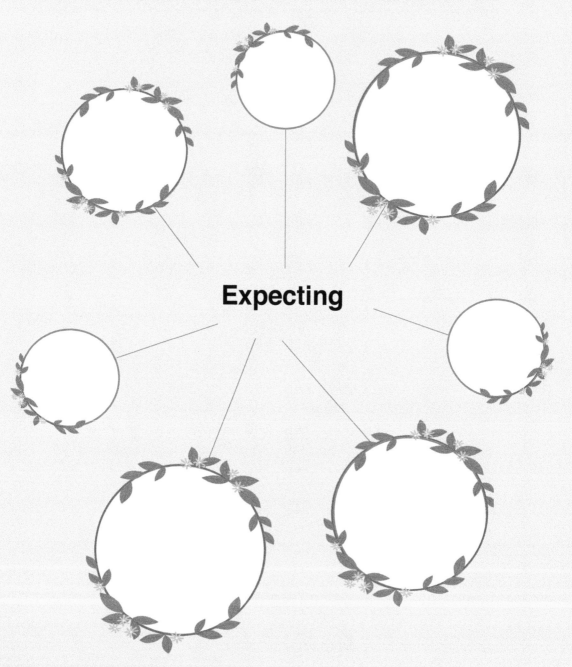

Expecting

Gravely Tired

Complete the crossword by filling in a word that fits each clue. Across are causes of pregnancy insomnia and down are remedies to help with third trimester pregnancy insomnia.

Across

1. A lot of anxiety
3. Don't go for the Joe
6. Cup size sensitivity
8. Knowledge gathered page by page
9. Achy stomach
10. Habits before sleeping
13. A mask, but for sound
15. No night hydration
16. Bringing on the heartache
17. A stuffed addition to your bed
18. Manual muscle relaxant
19. Baby pressing on bladder causes this

Down

2. You might pant
4. Concern
5. Sensible evening meal
7. Rich in long chains of amino acids
11. Bright REM
12. Write it down
14. The cost of holding up a heavy uterus

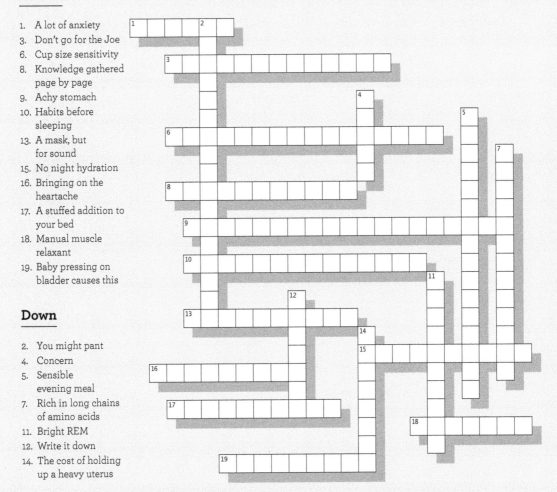

TIPS FOR THIRD TRIMESTER SYMPTOMS

Here are a few symptoms that might start happening as you're nearing the end of your pregnancy. As always, the easiest way to avoid many symptoms is to stay hydrated.

Shortness of Breath

The growing pressure of the uterus on your diaphragm can make it feel like it's tough to breathe. On top of that, progesterone lets the brain know to expand the lungs to take in more air while your body is growing a baby, but this can feel like you can't take a deep enough breath. What to do about it? Slow down. If you're feeling short of breath or winded, take it easy and make sure you're practicing good posture.

Frequent Urination

Toward the end of pregnancy, though, the baby has moved lower and can press on the bladder, causing even more frequent trips to the restroom. You also might find yourself with a little leak once in a while, especially after a laugh, a cough, or a sneeze. Though there isn't much you can do about moving the baby away from your bladder, you can wear a panty liner in case of leaks. Of course, if you feel a constant trickle or a sudden gush of fluid, call your doctor. That could be your water breaking!

Swollen Ankles

While sudden swelling around the face can be cause for concern, swelling around the feet and ankles is a pretty typical woe for expecting mamas. Pressure from the uterus and excess fluid can lead to swelling called edema, especially after a long day or in warmer weather. To help reduce swelling, elevate your feet when possible, avoid standing for long periods of time, and try not to cross your legs when sitting.

Hemorrhoids and Varicose Veins

Due to the increase in blood volume during pregnancy and the pressure a growing uterus can put on blood vessels, varicose veins are one of the unwelcome guests that can accompany pregnancy. Usually painless and harmless, these veins that swell over the surface of the skin can appear anywhere on the lower half of your body. Typically, we notice varicose veins on our legs, but hemorrhoids are actually just swollen veins that show up around the rectum. Elevate your feet when possible, sleep on your left side to keep blood flowing, and get moving.

Big Belly Blues

Put your puzzle-solving skills to the test with our third trimester common symptoms word scramble.

ivvid ademsr ＿ ＿ ＿ ＿ ＿ ＿ ＿ ＿ ＿ ＿ ＿

akbc npai ＿ ＿ ＿ ＿ ＿ ＿ ＿ ＿

maondlbia irtdfosomc ＿ ＿ ＿ ＿ ＿ ＿ ＿ ＿ ＿

＿ ＿ ＿ ＿ ＿ ＿ ＿ ＿ ＿

iuraonnit yfqentrule ＿ ＿ ＿ ＿ ＿ ＿ ＿ ＿ ＿ ＿

＿ ＿ ＿ ＿ ＿ ＿ ＿ ＿

lge cspmar ＿ ＿ ＿ ＿ ＿ ＿ ＿ ＿ ＿

hosnesrts of ebrhta ＿ ＿ ＿ ＿ ＿ ＿ ＿ ＿ ＿ ＿

＿ ＿ ＿ ＿ ＿

rssest ＿ ＿ ＿ ＿ ＿ ＿

htubrnare ＿ ＿ ＿ ＿ ＿ ＿ ＿ ＿ ＿

rwroy ＿ ＿ ＿ ＿ ＿

soceirav ievns ＿ ＿ ＿ ＿ ＿ ＿ ＿ ＿ ＿ ＿ ＿ ＿

tagieuf ＿ ＿ ＿ ＿ ＿ ＿ ＿

morehrioshd ＿ ＿ ＿ ＿ ＿ ＿ ＿ ＿ ＿ ＿

lowslen lkasen ＿ ＿ ＿ ＿ ＿ ＿ ＿ ＿ ＿ ＿ ＿ ＿

sonmaiin ＿ ＿ ＿ ＿ ＿ ＿ ＿ ＿

tnoxbra ckish ＿ ＿ ＿ ＿ ＿ ＿ ＿ ＿ ＿ ＿ ＿

Babymoon Planning

Ready to plan your babymoon? Narrow down your travel ideas by playing a fun little game of "Would You Rather?" Circle your favorite answers and ask your travel partner to circle theirs!

1. Would you rather spend more time **outside** or **inside**?

2. Would you rather be in a **swimsuit** or **cover it all up**?

3. Would you rather **sleep in and take naps** or **wake up early to experience something new**?

4. Would you rather **discover something new** or **be somewhere familiar**?

5. Would you rather **spend a little more** or **save a little more** on this trip?

6. Would you rather **eat a messy hot dog from a food truck on the go** or **slow down to enjoy candlelit dinner in a fine restaurant**?

7. Would you rather **take your time getting there** or **go as quickly as you can**?

8. Would you rather **stroll on a boardwalk in shorts** or **build a snowman after a snowfall**?

9. Would you rather **spend the night in a luxury hotel** or **camp in a tent**?

10. Would you rather **travel by train** or **by plane**?

PLANNING A BABYMOON

If you're the type of person who needs an excuse for a getaway, a pregnancy is the perfect one!

A babymoon is a little escape to get in one last uncomplicated trip with your partner. The next time you go on a vacation, you'll have to think about packing diapers and extra blankets and, of course, the burbling, wiggly carry-on that lived inside you for nine months!

Let's talk though a few tips for planning one last child-free getaway.

Time it.
Toward the end of the second trimester and into the beginning of the third is a great time to plan a babymoon. You're probably past the morning sickness, and you probably have more energy.

Keep your doctor in the loop.
As long as you're experiencing a normal, healthy pregnancy, your doctor is usually happy to sign off on a vacation. It's important to keep your medical provider in the loop and see if they have any special instructions for you.

Travel time.
When looking at places to go, think about how long it will take to get there. Both road trips and flights are fine up until a certain point in your pregnancy, but you can't stay in one position for too long.

Decide on a location.
Check the Centers for Disease Control and Prevention for any travel restrictions if you're going abroad, and also check with the airline or cruise line you're considering for any pregnancy-related restrictions.

Be prepared.
It's not the fun part of vacation planning, but it's best to look up the hospitals in the area ahead of time and make sure to bring along your insurance card and any other pertinent information, just in case.

Have fun.
Most importantly, this is a time to relax and reconnect with your partner and yourself. Let go of the worries that may have been on your mind and enjoy this vacation!

Maternal Instinct

How many six letter words can you make using the letters in MATERNITY?

_____   _____

_____   _____

_____   _____

_____   _____

_____   _____

_____   _____

_____   _____

_____   _____

_____   _____

_____   _____

_____   _____

_____   _____

_____   _____

_____   _____

_____   _____

_____   _____

_____   _____

Heartburn Help

Especially in the third trimester, your growing uterus is pressing up on the intestines and stomach. Use these clues to find remedies for that oh-so-annoying heartburn.

Across

1. Sweet aged dairy
5. Opposite of under + opposite of fasting
7. No room to move + covering for the body
9. Pulp fruit that you can juice
11. Sourced from cows
12. Little + Sit at the dinner table for these

Down

2. Red-haired nickname
3. Bubbles for your drink
4. Raise your gaze
6. A substance to neutralize acid
8. Legal stimulant in a cup
10. Sugar and _____ and everything nice

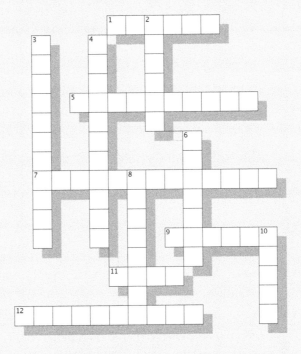

WHY HEARTBURN?

Even if you've never had heartburn before pregnancy, it's a common complaint and likely that you'll experience it at some point while expecting. Heartburn doesn't have anything to do with the heart. It's caused by stomach acid backing up into your esophagus, causing a burning sensation in your chest and throat. During pregnancy, your digestion slows down, giving food and acids more time in the stomach. At the same time, the hormones preparing your body for labor can also cause the band of muscle at the top of your stomach to relax. That allows acids from the stomach to flow back up into your esophagus. The growing bump pushing on your stomach doesn't help, either.

Thankfully, there are things that can help, and there's an end in sight.

Don't lie down immediately after eating. Try eating smaller, more frequent meals so that you don't overfill your stomach. Steer clear of spicy, acidic, and fatty foods.

Selecting a Pediatrician Checklist

Selecting a pediatrician early is necessary, because your baby will need their own doctor right away, even while you're both still in the hospital after birth! Here are some important questions to consider when you check out their offices. Use this checklist to record the doctor's responses and be sure to check off the questions as you go:

- ☐ If the need arises for your child to be hospitalized, where would he or she be admitted?

- ☐ What hospitals is the doctor associated with?

- ☐ Is the pediatrician's office conveniently located?

- ☐ Do the office hours work with your schedule?

- ☐ Are there evening or weekend hours?

- ☐ Do they have a separate waiting area for well children and sick children?

- ☐ Is the office staff friendly?

- ☐ Do you feel rushed in the office, either by the staff or the doctor?

- ☐ Do they seem to operate in an efficient manner?

- ☐ Is the office clean?

- ☐ Is there a nurse in the office who can answer routine questions?

- ☐ How does the doctor handle phone calls?

- ☐ When the pediatrician is on vacation or otherwise unavailable, who covers for them?

- ☐ Does the doctor have any specialties? What's the protocol if your baby needs to see a specialist?

- ☐ What is the office policy regarding the processing of insurance forms?

- ☐ What are the fees for different types of visits?

- ☐ Are there tests or bloodwork that can be done in-house?

Pregnancy Relief from A to Z

Pregnant women should always check with their doctor about taking any medications during a pregnancy. But if you get a little sick, there are over-the-counter meds that your doctor should agree are safe. Check out this list and see if you can find each of these OTC drugs in the word search!

Pain Relief:
Tylenol

Acetamino-phen

Digestive Upsets:
Antacids

Simethicone

Imodium
(after the first trimester)

Colds:
Robitussin

Cough drops

Vaporub

Allergies:
Chlor-Trimeton

Saline spray

Claritin

Constipation:
Fiber

Colace

Tucks

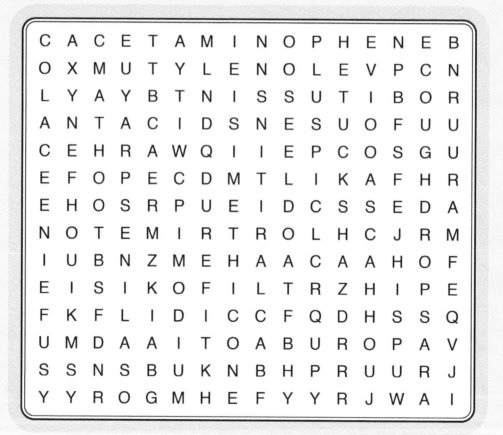

C A C E T A M I N O P H E N E B
O X M U T Y L E N O L E V P C N
L Y A Y B T N I S S U T I B O R
A N T A C I D S N E S U O F U U
C E H R A W Q I I E P C O S G U
E F O P E C D M T L I K A F H R
E H O S R P U E I D C S S E D A
N O T E M I R T R O L H C J R M
I U B N Z M E H A A C A A H O F
E I S I K O F I L T R Z H I P E
F K F L I D I C C F Q D H S S Q
U M D A A I T O A B U R O P A V
S S N S B U K N B H P R U U R J
Y Y R O G M H E F Y Y R J W A I

THE COMMON COLD, PREGNANCY REMIX

The common cold is especially common during pregnancy, though not all stuffy noses mean you've caught a cold. Stuffiness can happen often because the increase in blood flow to your mucus membranes causes swelling, including in the nose.

To determine if the stuffiness is really a cold, look to see if you've got other symptoms. Lots of sneezing, a sore or scratchy throat, a dry cough, or a fever can tip you off that it's more than swollen membranes.

There is a reason that you're more vulnerable to the common cold. Your immune system is suppressed and runs a little slower when you're expecting. Though it sounds bad, it's for a good reason: Your baby is a foreign entity. But making your body more hospitable for your baby also makes you more susceptible to cold and flu viruses.

There are plenty of natural remedies and ways to deal with a cold and ease your symptoms. Plenty of rest and fluids will be your best friend. And what better excuse for long afternoon naps than pregnancy and a cold?

If you're not feeling up to chugging water, try warm drinks like ginger tea or even sip on chicken noodle soup. Just don't let yourself get dehydrated. It's important to drink fluids when you're sick under normal circumstances; it's even more important when you're pregnant.

A saline spray or mist can help soothe your nasal passages, and a cool mist humidifier is great for keeping the air moist. Saltwater gargles and honey are both safe ways to treat a sore throat as well.

In most cases, a cold will pass in a couple of weeks. If your cold lasts longer than two weeks, talk to your doctor if you haven't already. And of course, if you ever develop a fever, call your doctor.

Baby Shower Checklist

Your baby shower is a milestone in your pregnancy and helps you get ready for your baby's arrival. A shower allows your friends and family to shower you and your wee one with love and gifts. Ideally, you'll receive many of the things you'll need for baby's arrival. Use the prompts and the checklist to keep your shower plans organized!

Who will host your shower? _____

What is your idea for a theme or color scheme? _____

When should your shower happen (date/time)? _____

Where would you like it to take place? _____

Have you determined a budget? _____

Checklist:

- ☐ Complete registry
- ☐ Finalize guest list
- ☐ Create invitations (online or printed)
- ☐ Organize food
- ☐ Order dessert (cake or cupcakes are classic)
- ☐ Take care of drinks (a signature shower drink is a fun idea!)
- ☐ Get tableware

- ☐ Select decorations
- ☐ Choose shower games
- ☐ Arrange for game prizes
- ☐ Create a music playlist
- ☐ Shop for party favors
- ☐ Assign a photographer
- ☐ Designate someone to take notes on the gifts for thank you notes later
- ☐ Pick a shower outfit

Nursery Essentials

When it comes down to it, all the furniture that you really need for your baby is a place for them to lay their head. But by now that nesting phase has probably kicked in and you're feeling like you need it ALL. Let's see what you need and what items you can get by without. Look for and circle the words hidden in the puzzle.

Baby nursery essentials:

Crib

Mattress

Nursing chair

Changing pad

Monitor

Bedding

What you can do without:

Mobile

Changing table

Nightlight

Toys

Wipe warmer

```
A  B  S  S  E  R  T  T  A  M  O  I  U  M
Q  R  O  S  O  U  Y  A  F  S  K  G  W  T
E  M  Q  N  I  G  H  T  L  I  G  H  T  M
U  E  U  C  E  A  T  Q  H  Y  C  O  S  U
N  U  R  S  I  N  G  C  H  A  I  R  S  E
D  A  P  G  N  I  G  N  A  H  C  I  I  M
W  I  P  E  W  A  R  M  E  R  C  E  I  O
B  E  D  D  I  N  G  I  M  U  A  E  R  B
I  O  J  A  O  B  I  R  C  U  P  B  J  I
G  D  U  M  O  C  M  W  E  T  O  Y  S  L
C  H  A  N  G  I  N  G  T  A  B  L  E  E
J  B  M  O  N  I  T  O  R  N  A  H  W  J
```

Nesting Checklist

A nesting mama is a force of nature. Here's a few classic items to tackle with all of this newfound energy. Unscramble these words and let's see what you've already crossed off your list!

☐ llastni rcetasa __ __ __ __ __ __ __ __ __ __ __ __ __

☐ hswa ybba scotleh __ __ __ __ __ __ __ __ __ __ __ __ __ __

☐ kapc phsioatl gba __ __ __ __ __ __ __ __ __ __ __ __ __ __

☐ idbul bric __ __ __ __ __ __ __ __ __

☐ zeefre slema __ __ __ __ __ __ __ __ __ __

☐ sawh wsniowd __ __ __ __ __ __ __ __ __ __ __

☐ spele __ __ __ __ __

☐ pewi brebaodsas __ __ __ __ __ __ __ __ __ __ __ __ __

☐ eceudrttl __ __ __ __ __ __ __ __ __

☐ ehedscul bslli __ __ __ __ __ __ __ __ __ __ __ __ __

☐ ahsw nbdiged __ __ __ __ __ __ __ __ __ __ __

☐ anelc raepcst __ __ __ __ __ __ __ __ __ __ __

☐ ucst nasf __ __ __ __ __ __ __ __

☐ skcot reaidsp __ __ __ __ __ __ __ __ __ __ __

☐ nreazogi cltoses __ __ __ __ __ __ __ __ __ __ __ __ __ __

PREPARE YOUR PETS

Your pet most likely already has an idea of what's going on, or at least knows that things are changing. Many pets do just fine without any preparation before baby comes home. But if your animal companion has been your "baby" up until this point, it's wise to start slowly introducing them to your new shared life.

Introduce Sounds

Start using some of the items that your baby will use when you bring them home. Turn on a toy, play the white noise. You could even find some baby crying noises and play them for your pet. It's not something you'll need to do constantly, but the key is to introduce them now so it's not totally disorienting when your baby arrives.

Introduce Smells

Both dogs and cats experience much of their world through scent, and though you don't have your newborn for them to smell yet, baby items come with quite a few new aromas. Try to prepare for the baby with your pet present so they can get used to these new smells.

Introduce Emotional Changes

If your fur baby is used to having all of your attention, ignore them once in a while, or let someone else take care of them. Once you have a newborn, your priorities will shift away from your pet, so start easing them into a new groove.

Introduce New Rules

If you're going to have boundaries or rules when baby comes, like no pets in the crib or bassinet, start enforcing them now.

Introduce Them to Babies

If there's someone in your life with their own wee one, plan a play date so your fur baby can experience the sounds and smells that come along with a baby. Another option is to walk around with a swaddle or other baby items in your hands as though you are holding a baby. Let your pet see you caring for something else.

Introduce Them to Your Baby

When the time comes, it's okay to love on your fur baby along with your new baby! Let them sit with you when you nurse, talk to them both when changing diapers, or pet them while you cuddle baby. It might be a great way to let them start their own bond. Just don't leave your pet and your baby together without supervision.

Delivery Room Match

You'll encounter many items throughout labor and delivery. Place each item where it belongs by using the words at the top and writing them in the box at the bottom with the matching professional/person.

Cup of Ice

Extra Pillow

Stethoscope

Wheelchair

Blankets

Meals

Pain Medications

Prescription Pad

Amniotic Hook

Forceps

Scissors

Speculum

Laparoscopic Sponges

Sutures

Vacuum

Hemostat

Camera

Light Box

Memory Card

Tripod

Flash

Pose

Slippers

Robe

Contractions

Glow

Holding Baby

Diaper

Pacifier

Onesie

Mittens

Hat

Swaddle

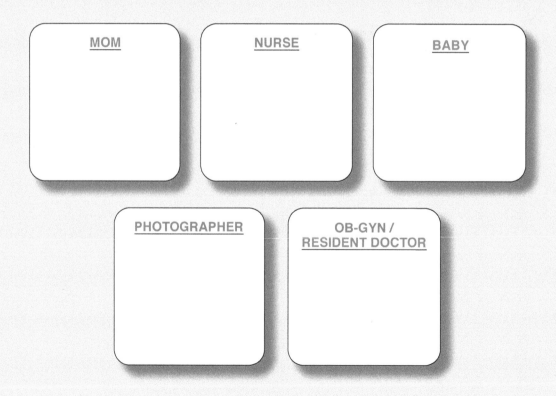

MOM

NURSE

BABY

PHOTOGRAPHER

OB-GYN /
RESIDENT DOCTOR

Nesting Madness

The urge to clean just about everything will hit you hard during a pregnancy. While you're cleaning up and clearing out every nook and cranny around you, make a note of it! Write the craziest thing you've done in the name of "nesting":

I threw away _____

I wiped down our _____

I washed the _____

I organized _____

I vacuumed _____

I shampooed _____

I cleaned out _____

I replaced _____

I sorted through _____

I decluttered the _____

I used a _____

Two as One

During pregnancy, the two of you operate as a team of one.

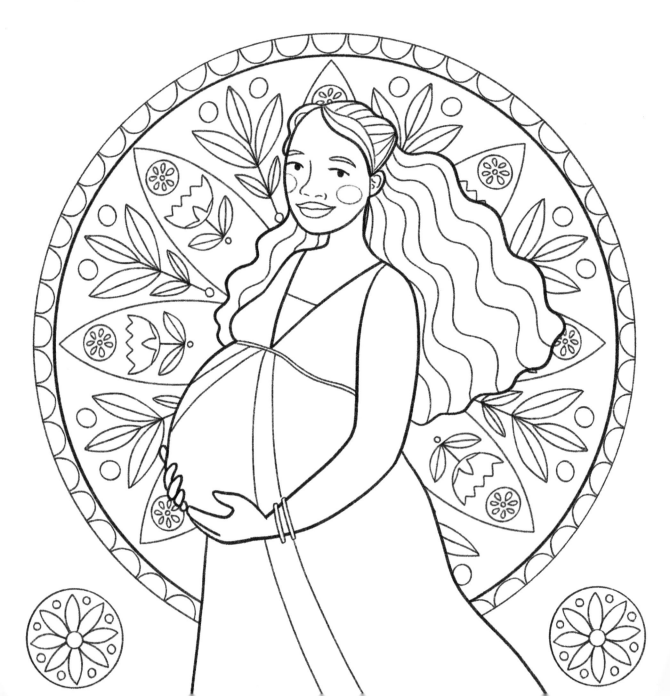

This or That: Pink or Blue Edition

A gender reveal party can be a fun way to surprise your friends and family—and yourself—with a sweet revelation about your baby. Read through the This or That list and circle your favorites from each line to help you choose a method for the big reveal.

cake **VS** cupcake

balloons **VS** silly string

smoke **VS** powder

piñata party **VS** opening a box

spell it out **VS** sibling signs

paint splatter **VS** confetti popper

car exhaust **VS** color-filled ball

ice cream **VS** bubble gum

cotton candy **VS** cookies

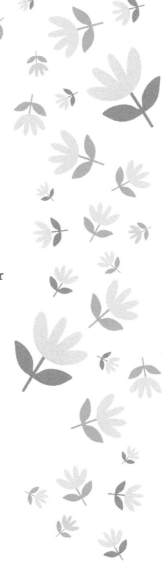

My Water Broke!

Write down the first word that first comes to mind when you read these parts of speech. Then read the story aloud using the words from your list. Try reading this aloud with a partner.

NOUN 1 _____

ADJECTIVE 1 _____

ADJECTIVE 2 _____

ADJECTIVE 3 _____

PLACE _____

ONE OF THE FIVE SENSES _____

_____

ADJECTIVE 4 _____

ADJECTIVE 5 _____

VERB 1 (ending in -ing) _____

_____

VERB 2 _____

ADJECTIVE 6 _____

ADVERB (ending in -ly) _____

_____

NOUN 2 _____

ADJECTIVE 7 _____

VERB 3 (ending in -ed) _____

VERB 4 (ending in -ed) _____

ADJECTIVE 8 _____

COLOR _____

VERB 5 (ending in -ed) _____

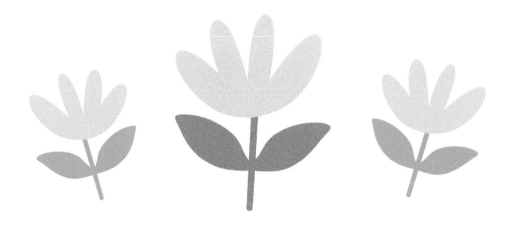

Once upon a _____ there was a[n] _____ woman who was
　　　　　　　 NOUN 1　　　　　　　　 ADJECTIVE 1

nine months pregnant. Even though it seemed like she had to pee every five

minutes, she decided to go to her friend's wedding at a[n] _____ hall
　　　　　　　　　　　　　　　　　　　　　　　　　　　　　 ADJECTIVE 2

on the campus of their alma mater, _____ School of _____
　　　　　　　　　　　　　　　　　 ADJECTIVE 3 (PLACE)　　　　　 ONE OF THE FIVE

_____. At the end of the ceremony, the officiant sternly said that if anyone
SENSES

objected to this union, they should speak now or forever hold their peace.

Right then a[n] _____ pain struck her _____ belly, which was
　　　　　　　　 ADJECTIVE 4　　　　　　　　　 ADJECTIVE 5

_____ . I _____ a[n] _____ squeal and
　 VERB 1 (ending in -ing)　　 VERB 2　　　　　 ADJECTIVE 5

everyone in the place turned _____ to see her standing in a[n]
　　　　　　　　　　　　　　 ADVERB (ending in -ly)

_____ 2 of water. Her water had broken. The entire room _____
ADJECTIVE 6 NOUN　　　　　　　　　　　　　　　　　　　　　　　　　　 VERB 3

_____ as she _____ her husband's hand and
(ending in -ed)　　　　　　　 VERB 4 (ending in -ed)

yelled, "We are having a baby!" Her face went _____. Between
　　　　　　　　　　　　　　　　　　　　　 ADJECTIVE 7 (COLOR)

contractions she _____ and apologized over and over as
　　　　　　　　　 VERB 5 (ending in -ed)

the ambulance arrived. It was the only kind of dramatic wedding upstaging a

bride and groom couldn't help but enjoy.

Who's Your Baby?

Your baby is so close and yet so far away! Take this quiz to get a peek at the little one you're about to meet for the first time.

1. **At the end of the seventh month, about how long is your baby?**
   A. 23 inches
   B. 30 inches
   C. 14 inches
   D. 50 inches

2. **Near the end of the seventh month, what's being deposited on your baby?**
   A. Fat
   B. Moles
   C. Freckles
   D. Skin pigment

3. **Near the end of the seventh month, your baby has fully developed _____.**
   A. Smell
   B. Taste
   C. Hearing
   D. Touch

4. **In the eighth month, you may notice baby _____ more.**
   A. Moving
   B. Kicking
   C. Having bowel movements
   D. Sneezing

5. **What part of the baby's body develops rapidly during the eighth month?**
   A. Brain
   B. Feet
   C. Heart
   D. Lungs

6. **What organ is still immature around the eighth month?**
   A. Stomach
   B. Eyes
   C. Lungs
   D. Liver

7. **At end of the third trimester, your baby can** _____.

   A. Close their eyes

   B. Turn their head

   C. Grasp firmly

   D. All of the above

8. **At the end of the third trimester, most babies will begin to get in position for labor and delivery.**

   T / F

9. **At the end of ninth month, how long is your baby?**

   A. 12 to 14 inches

   B. 14 to 16 inches

   C. 16 to 18 inches

   D. 14 inches from crown to rump

10. **Ideally, which way should your baby be facing for delivery?**

    A. Sideways across your belly.

    B. Head down

    C. Feet down

    D. It doesn't matter.

Registry Checklist

Use the vowels to complete the list and build your registry checklist with all of the essentials!

Vowels: A E I O U

T __ B

W __ SH

CR __ B SH __ __ TS

P __ J __ M __ S

S __ CKS

__ N __ S __ __ S

BL __ NK __ TS

SW __ DDL __ RS

B __ RP CL __ THS

B __ BS

D __ __ P __ R P __ __ L

D __ __ P __ RS

W __ P __ S

D __ __ P __ R CR __ __ M

BR __ __ ST P __ MP

CR __ B M __ TR __ SS

N __ RS __ NG P __ LL __ W

B __ TTL __ S

H __ GH CH __ __ R

N __ __ L TR __ MM __ R

TH __ RM __ M __ T __ R

CR __ B

R __ CK __ NG CH __ __ R

CH __ NG __ NG T __ BL __

B __ BY M __ N __ T __ R

T __ __ THER

C __ RS __ __ T

STR __ LL __ R

B __ BY C __ RR __ __ R

D __ __ P __ R B __ G

PL __ Y Y __ RD

The Waddle Workout

Thanks to all of those crazy changes in your body, just about everything you do in the third trimester is a workout. Unscramble the words for a list of things that could totally count as a workout when you're nearing the end of pregnancy.

yignt sceoehals __ __ __ __ __ __ __ __ __ __ __ __ __ __

lgnoirl revo __ __ __ __ __ __ __ __ __ __

ndsintga pu __ __ __ __ __ __ __ __ __ __

awnklig __ __ __ __ __ __ __

cnigblmi rssiat __ __ __ __ __ __ __ __ __ __ __ __ __

egtbhainr __ __ __ __ __ __ __ __ __

pinizpg tpnsa __ __ __ __ __ __ __ __ __ __ __

aihsgvn egsl __ __ __ __ __ __ __ __ __ __

tegnai __ __ __ __ __ __

naintpgi letosina __ __ __ __ __ __ __ __ __ __ __ __ __ __

kgilatn __ __ __ __ __ __ __

Take It or Leave It!

People love to give their two cents when you're pregnant. You'll hear everything from ridiculous medical opinions from strangers to wonderful parenting tips from old friends or relatives. Here are two columns: One is for the good advice you've heard and want to remember, and one is for the things people have said that you're going to laugh about later.

TAKE IT   LEAVE IT

_____   _____

_____   _____

_____   _____

_____   _____

_____   _____

_____   _____

_____   _____

_____   _____

_____   _____

_____   _____

_____   _____

_____   _____

Third Trimester Checklist

The third trimester is when things seem to simultaneously speed up and slow down. This is the time you'll have more appointments, so make sure to ask all of your questions so that you're feeling confident and ready! Check off each item on the list as you make it through these last few weeks.

- ☐ Do a home safety check.
- ☐ Start fetal kick counts.
- ☐ Write up your birth plan.
- ☐ Enjoy your baby shower.
- ☐ Send baby shower thank you notes for gifts.
- ☐ Take a childbirth class—and a breastfeeding class, if you want to.
- ☐ Talk to your baby.
- ☐ If you want to do cord-blood banking, order a kit.
- ☐ Stock the freezer.
- ☐ Buy any baby items you still need.
- ☐ Prepare a baby first aid kit and stock the medicine cabinet.
- ☐ Finish setting up the nursery.
- ☐ Install a car seat and get it inspected.

- ☐ Pack your hospital bag.
- ☐ Pre-register with the hospital.
- ☐ Choose a pediatrician.
- ☐ Do your group B strep test between weeks 35 and 37.
- ☐ If your doctor recommends it, take a nonstress test to check the baby's heart.
- ☐ If your doctor recommends it, do a biophysical profile to evaluate your baby's health.
- ☐ Wash baby's clothes and bedding.
- ☐ Arrange for people to help you after the birth.
- ☐ Get a few nursing tops or nightgowns if you're planning to breastfeed.
- ☐ Have your house cleaned.

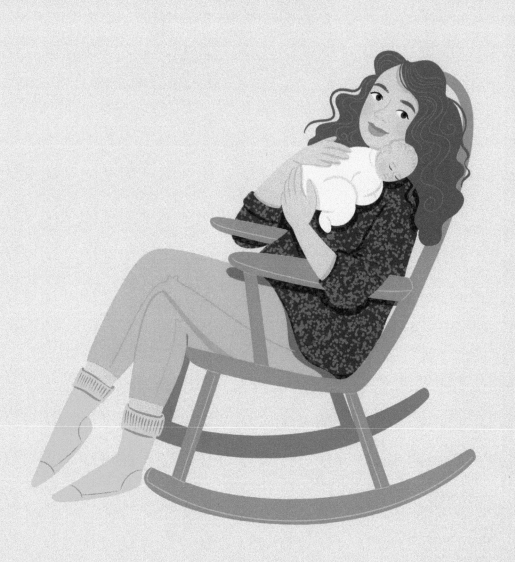

Childbirth

Labor of Love

Going through labor is painful and beautiful and a total adrenaline rush. To help you remember it later, write down some memories of labor. Most of the prompts will apply to most women, but feel free to skip any that don't apply to you.

When I started feeling contractions, I felt _____

_____ .

The first thing I did when I knew I was starting labor was _____

_____ .

I called my doctor when _____

_____ .

I grabbed my go-bag and traveled to the hospital by _____

_____ .

When the staff checked me into a temporary room to check labor signs, I saw ___

_____ .

A nurse checked my dilation, and I felt _____

_____ .

My blood was drawn and my blood pressure was being monitored. And when my

baby's heart and my contractions were being monitored, I knew _____

_____ .

Once labor was confirmed, I moved into a room that was _____

_____.

Referring to my birth plan made me feel _____

_____.

The pain management I used during labor was _____

_____.

There were a lot of medical staff coming in and out of the room, and I felt _____

_____.

When I was ready to start pushing, the hospital staff shifted my room into a

delivery room, and I felt _____

_____.

The most surprising thing about labor was _____

_____.

When I held my baby for the first time, I felt _____

_____.

ON A NEED TO KNOW BASIS

An informed mama is a calm mama! Labor can already bring enough curveballs. Here's a primer on what you need to know.

There's only one definitive sign of labor.
Every woman's body is different, and you can't really predict how labor will go. Your water might break on its own, or it might not. You might have a "bloody show," which is when you lose your mucus plug, or you might not. But you can count on having contractions. If you're experiencing regular contractions, you're in labor!

If you're in early labor, take it easy.
It might sound counterintuitive to rest, and your first reaction may be to run about in a fury while frantically gathering your belongings! But take a beat. You don't know how long your labor might last, and in the early stages when contractions are still irregular, it's best to get rest while you can.

If you're starting to go into labor at home, eat!
If you're in early labor and you haven't had "5-1-1" contractions—minute-long contractions happening every five minutes for an hour—make sure you eat BEFORE checking into the hospital. While there are some exceptions, most hospitals won't allow you to eat while you're in active labor, and some will allow only ice chips. Birthing centers are different, so ask ahead of time.

Accept that your birth plan may go out the window.
Preparation for labor and delivery is important, but things will not always happen just like you planned. It's okay! Sometimes your medical providers will need to make changes to the plan, and sometimes you'll change your mind when you get into the thick of it. Because you don't know exactly what labor will be like for you, especially as a first-time mom, you may need to adapt to what works in the moment.

Be kind to yourself.
Just because delivering a baby is natural doesn't mean that it's easy. It can be chaotic, long, and difficult. The great news is that you can do hard things. The whole process is perfectly imperfect, and you're bringing life into this world. Be gentle with yourself. There's so much pressure on new moms to do things the "right" way, but the right way doesn't exist. You are doing what you can, and you are going to love your baby so much, and that is enough. You are enough. You're doing great.

Bring Baby Home!

Complete the maze to help the stork bring a little baby home!

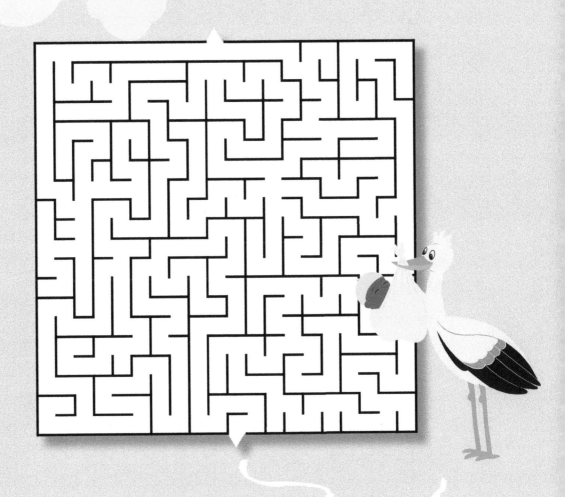

Baby Talk

Becoming a mom is a learning experience, and some of what you'll learn is a bunch of new words! How much of this new vocab do you know?

1. **What do you call a doctor who specializes in treating children?**
   A. Neurosurgeon
   B. Podiatrist
   C. Pediatrician
   D. Veterinarian

2. **What does NICU stand for?**
   A. Northern Ireland Cry University
   B. Nursery intensive crying unit
   C. North impressive casting unit
   D. Neonatal intensive care unit

3. **What is baby formula?**
   A. Powder specifically made for babies to drink from bottle.
   B. Baby race car
   C. Both A and B
   D. Dried milk

4. **What is C-section short for?**
   A. Section of Caesar salad
   B. Caesarean section
   C. A covert government agency.
   D. The best place to watch a football game in a dome.

5. **What is an epidural?**
   A. A hypodermic device used for emergency allergic reactions.
   B. A spiritual experience during childbirth.
   C. A pain inhibitor administered in the lower spine.
   D. Enduring childbirth without fainting.

6. **What is the APGAR score?**
   A. The total number of game apps on your phone.
   B. The circumference of your ankles at birth.
   C. The length of your linea negra.
   D. A test given to newborns soon after birth to see if extra medical attention is needed.

7. **What is a lactation consultant?**
   A. A specialist who helps you and your baby figure out nursing.
   B. Someone who helps if you have deficits in your budget.
   C. A person who aids in deciding your baby name.
   D. Someone who likes milk.

8. **What does neonatal mean?**

   A. Three kinds of babies

   B. National baby day

   C. Relating to newborn children

   D. Having to do with the nose

9. **What does the doctor mean if he says the baby is crowning?**

   A. The baby will grow up to be a king.

   B. The baby has hair shaped like a crown.

   C. The baby came out smiling

   D. The baby's head has fully emerged in the vagina during delivery.

10. **What does induction mean?**

   A. The process of bringing on childbirth that usually involves medication.

   B. A surgery for tear duct implants.

   C. A study of ductwork in a home.

   D. To be taken without permission.

THE BIRTH PLAN

Having a birth plan in place is a way for you to mentally prepare for childbirth. Writing down what you want and sharing it with your partner and doctor will ensure you're all on the same page. A birth plan is a list of your preferences for the big day so that everyone will know exactly what you want and your partner will be able to advocate for you.

Have you thought about who you want to be in the room with you? Do you have a certain way you would like to deliver? Do you want a water birth, a midwife-assisted birth, a C-section? Research here is important so you can make informed decisions. Start envisioning this special day early on. Once you have researched your options for labor and delivery and have a plan for what you want, it's time to write it all down.

There is no one way to create a birth plan, but it's important to keep it simple and to the point. Childbirth can be pretty chaotic, so you want your plan to be clear and concise.

The main goal of every childbirth is to deliver a healthy baby with minimal trauma to mama. The happier and more comfortable you are, the easier it will be for you! So, consider what will make YOU feel taken care of. This is a time where you'll be doing all the hard work, so plan it out according to your own preferences. No one else's opinion should matter.

Consider things like the atmosphere you want. Do you want the room quiet or filled with your own music? Do you want the lights dimmed? Do you want someone there to take photos? What pain management do you want? Do you want an epidural, or do you want to try other options like a warm shower or massage?

Once you've done some research, speak with your doctor. Bring a written birth plan along to one of your appointments and ask to review it together. Ask lots of questions. This is a huge medical event, and you want to be armed with information. You might want to discuss a plan B with your doctor in case plan A doesn't work.

Preparation is important, but flexibility is key! Remember that you chose your doctor for a reason, and in the end, it's important to trust their judgment. While there's a chance everything will go according to your plan, there's also a chance that it won't. What's most important is that you and your baby are healthy.

And remember to enjoy this remarkable time. Every woman's birth story is different, and it will be a special memory you can share with your little one.

Birth Plan Checklist

A birth plan is important to think about and write down ahead of time. Writing it down will prevent misunderstandings, and it'll help your partner and medical team advocate for your desires. Complete this checklist to help get you started on creating your own birth plan.

YES / NO QUESTIONS

☐ / ☐ Do you want your partner to aid in catching the baby at birth?

☐ / ☐ Do you want photos during birth?

☐ / ☐ Have you decided on the type of birth you're planning?

☐ / ☐ Are there specific birthing positions you'd like your doctor to assist?

☐ / ☐ Do you want to walk around during labor?

☐ / ☐ Do you have a preference on the use of Pitocin to speed labor?

☐ / ☐ Do you want pain medication that will ease labor pains?

☐ / ☐ Do you want a lot of visitors at the hospital after your baby is born?

☐ / ☐ Do you want a mirror so you can watch your baby being born?

☐ / ☐ Would you like to have your spouse or partner cut the umbilical cord?

☐ / ☐ If you have a boy, do you want him to be circumcised?

☐ / ☐ Do you want your baby to be given a pacifier?

☐ / ☐ Would you like to hold your baby skin-to-skin immediately after birth?

☐ / ☐ Do you have plans for breastfeeding?

☐ / ☐ Do you want to bring your own outfit to wear during your stay at the hospital?

☐ / ☐ Do you want to bring your own music for the hospital stay?

☐ / ☐ Would you like to have your favorite blankets or pillows?

THE HOME STRETCH: CHILDBIRTH CLASSES AND MATERNITY HOSPITAL TOURS

You have a ton on your plate in the third trimester, and it can be easy to skip over taking a hospital tour or a childbirth class as your schedule fills with appointments and baby prep. However, if you can find the time, you should really try to take a class and a tour. It will help you prepare for the big day.

Check with your hospital to see what classes they offer. They might host a childbirth class, like Lamaze, or a car seat safety class. There's plenty you can learn, and some of it is stuff you might not have even thought of. While you don't have to take any classes to have your baby, it can certainly help you feel prepped.

Out of all of the things you can schedule at the hospital, making sure you get a tour is important. You'll want to know where to park, which doors to enter, and where to go when you have to get to the maternity ward in a hurry. Think of the tour as a kind of emergency drill: You want to know what to do in advance so that, if you're panicking in the moment, you won't *also* panic about knowing which hallway you're going through.

You put a ton of energy and work into a pregnancy, and the hospital is where you'll have your grand finale. Being armed with as much information as possible will help you stay clearheaded when you're in labor. When you minimize the number of things to worry about, you'll have an easier time sticking to your birth plan.

There's no such thing as too many questions when you're on the hospital tour finding out where you'll be delivering your baby and what the rooms look like. Go in prepared to ask away, and leave feeling more prepared to have that sweet babe!

Here are 25 questions to have on your list:

1. Are the rooms all private or are some shared? Do I need to call in advance for a private room?

2. Are there fees for private rooms?

3. Do all of the rooms look like the one we're being shown? Are some smaller or otherwise different?

4. Will I be in one room during my entire stay, or is there a separate postpartum room?

5. Is there a television?

6. What happens if the labor and delivery rooms are all full?

7. Will there be access to a shower or birthing tub? Are these private or shared?

8. Am I allowed to walk around during labor?

9. Will I be allowed to eat or drink during labor?

10. What is your intervention rate here, meaning how often does labor involve medical procedures like episiotomies and C-sections?

11. Is this a teaching hospital? Do residents attend my labor or birth? Do they need my permission?

12. What are the situations that may take me away from my birth partner?

13. Is there Wi-Fi available?

14. Can my spouse sleep in my room? Are there accommodations for them?

15. When does the kitchen open and close?

16. Is there a NICU? Where is it located?

17. What happens when I arrive in labor? Where do I get checked for signs of labor?

18. Is there a limit to how many people are allowed in the delivery room?

19. Does the hospital have policies on photography or video equipment during labor and delivery?

20. What is your policy on baby care after birth? Will it be performed in my room or is the baby taken elsewhere?

21. Can my baby sleep in the room with me?

22. Do you offer lactation support?

23. What security measures are in place for my baby?

24. What are the visiting hours? Are there age restrictions for visitors?

25. Is there a certain time of day for a standard discharge?

Babe in Arms

Color this little babe as you dream of all the special momentsyou'll have holding your own!

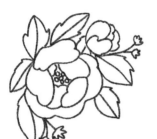
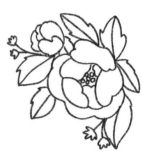
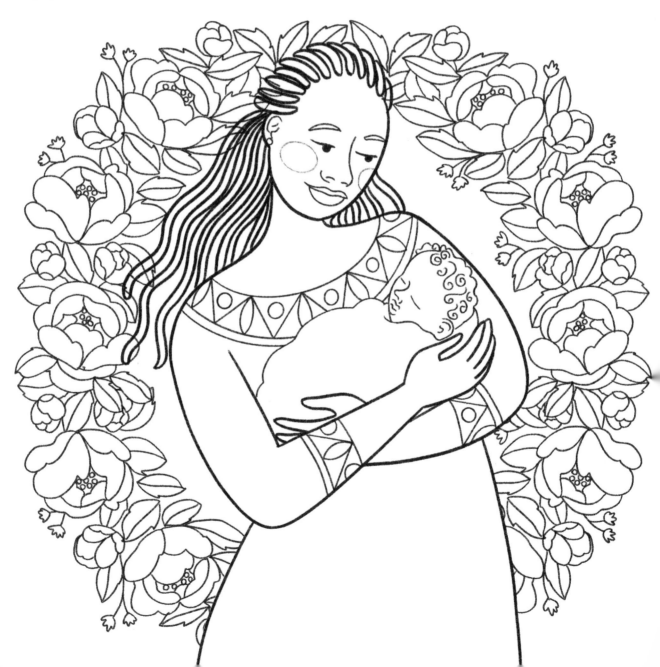

Baby's First Stuff

Find and circle the words listed here, which are all newborn essentials to bring to the hospital! Look for them in all directions, including backward and diagonally.

Car seat

Onesie

Hat

Mittens

Swaddle

Blanket

Pacifier

Socks

Diaper bag

Diapers

Wipes

Burp cloths

Nursing pillow

Name

```
Z N K Y A D S P N X U J G B E
S U C S H S E P I W N N A E R
K R I R W N M I T T N C B N S
W S S E S N T H O E H F R A H
I I E P W I P A C B O S E C T
P N F A A B U T L P N C P S O
T G D I D E S A A E A O A K L
N P P D D E N C T R A N I C C
A I T M L K I T S T P E D O P
M L N A E F I E C T C S L S R
E L E T I M A M Y Y R I P W U
U O W E D T L P C P O E N F B
D W R R U M E K P R E I W F F
```

Mama Match

Fill in the blanks with a synonym from the box.

1. Push _____

2. Contraction _____

3. Heartbeat _____

4. Fluid _____

5. Lamaze _____

6. Doctor _____

7. Nurse _____

8. Cry _____

9. Joy _____

10. Swaddle _____

11. Labor _____

12. Hospital _____

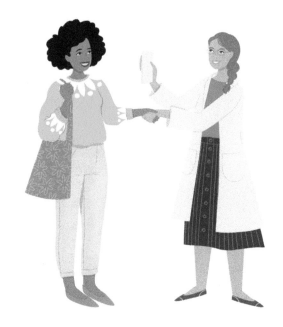

SYNONYMS:

Infirmary	Sheathe	Work	Breathing Techniques
Howling	Thrust	Pulsation	
Aqueous	Physician	Tightening	Caretaker
			Bliss

Expanding CONTRACTIONS

How many eight letter words can you make using the letters in
CONTRACTIONS?

_____   _____

_____   _____

_____   _____

_____   _____

_____   _____

_____   _____

_____   _____

_____   _____

_____   _____

_____   _____

_____   _____

_____   _____

_____   _____

_____   _____

_____   _____

_____   _____

EPIDURAL: TO NUMB OR NOT TO NUMB?

Epidural anesthesia is a form of pain management for labor and delivery. Epidurals are the most popular method for fast relief. According to the American Pregnancy Association, medical providers give this form of pain relief to more than 50 percent of women giving birth in hospitals.

What is it?

An epidural is a regional anesthesia that numbs the lower half of your body. It's intentionally a pain *reliever* and not a full anesthesia—you need some feeling to push. It causes numbness, which reduces the pain of contractions and pushing.

How do I get it?

An epidural is typically administered when you're dilated to about four or five centimeters, about halfway through labor. However, the timing may vary depending on your doctor and the specifics of your birth. If you choose an epidural, an anesthesiologist will be called to administer a small needle and catheter into your lower back (after numbing the area first, of course). Typically, you feel only some pressure on your back or spinal area when an epidural is being administered. You should feel relief within 20 minutes.

Will it help with labor?

Every woman's body is different, so every woman responds to an epidural a little differently. Some women love having an epidural. For others, an epidural can make pushing more difficult. There can also be some serious side effects, so talk with your doctor about the risks while you're finalizing your birth plan. If you do get an epidural, communicate with your medical team if you're feeling uncomfortable, and they'll help you work through it.

Baby's First Playlist

When creating a playlist(s) for the hospital, think about the different moments you'll experience. You might want a calming playlist for early stages when you need to rest and relax, a motivating playlist to give you the energy to push through, and a joyful playlist for later on when you're holding your sweet babe.

Song that best describes motherhood _____

Song that best describes my pregnancy _____

Song that I sing to my baby _____

Song that helps me breathe _____

Song that calms me _____

Song that always makes me smile _____

Song that always makes me cry (joyful tears) _____

Song that makes me feel like dancing with my partner _____
_____

Song that inspires me not to give up _____

Song that comes to mind when thinking of the word PUSH _____
_____

Song that I remember from my own childhood _____
_____

My favorite love song _____

A fun song with the word "baby" in it _____

My favorite lullaby _____

Postpartum Recovery Smoothie

MAKES: 20 OUNCES | **PREP TIME:** 5 MINUTES

Breastfeeding can be that sweet bonding time you've dreamt of, so don't give up at the first sign of trouble. There are some foods that aid in healing your body and boost milk supply, so whip up this smoothie to kick-start the postpartum recovery process!

1 cup coconut water

½ cup spinach

1 serving vanilla protein powder (according to package)

1 serving collagen powder (according to package)

1 teaspoon bee pollen

1 serving MCT oil (according to package)

½ cup rolled oats (uncooked)

1 cup frozen tropical fruit (for flavor)

1 banana (optional)

Toss all ingredients in a blender and blend until smooth. Pour in a glass and enjoy!

TIP: Any kind of oats will work, but I've found that rolled oats and quick oats make for a creamier smoothie.

Nursing Bliss

The best tip for nursing your baby is to stay calm. They can feel your energy!
Now is the perfect time to practice as you color in this page of sweet nursing bliss.

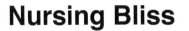

Go-Bag Go-Time

When you're headed to the hospital, you're in for one of the hardest, craziest things your body has ever accomplished. Solve the clues and fill in the crossword puzzle with things you might want to bring in your go-bag.

Across

4. Pit perfume
9. Bound pages
11. Something to eat between meals
12. A way to hear tunes
13. Handheld detangler

Down

1. A cleaning tool for your pearly whites
2. Colorful pages to turn in a monthly subscription form
3. Nighttime head rest
5. Appendage warmers sometimes made into puppets
6. Over-the-shoulder mom bosom holder
7. Moisturize your kisser
8. Be careful not to fall in these
10. Ponytail holder anyone?
14. Article of clothing fit for a king

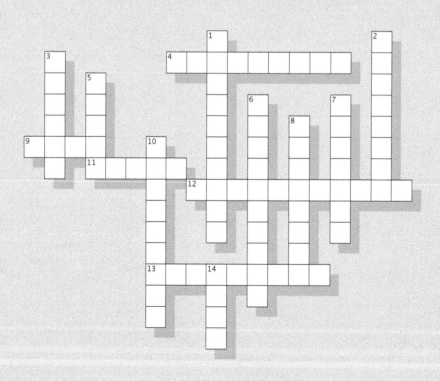

Delivering from DELIVERY

How many six letter words can you make using the letters in DELIVERY?

_____   _____

_____   _____

_____   _____

_____   _____

_____   _____

_____   _____

_____   _____

_____   _____

_____   _____

_____   _____

_____   _____

_____   _____

_____   _____

_____   _____

_____   _____

_____   _____

EVICTION NOTICE: THE OVERDUE BABY

Feeling uncomfortable that your due date has come and gone and you're ready to hand over an eviction notice? If only it were that simple!

While the due date is set at 40 weeks, you're not "officially" overdue until you've passed 42 weeks. Most women give birth between 38 and 42 weeks, and there isn't a particular reason that some babies like to stay in utero a little longer.

If you begin to pass your due date, your doctor will keep an eye on you. If you desire, some doctors will intervene after week 41, and you can schedule a time to induce labor. Delivering more than two weeks past your due date can carry some risks, and most doctors will urge intervention at that point.

Midwives typically take more of a "wait and see" approach. A midwife will generally wait until 42 weeks before suggesting intervention.

While there are some folk wisdom methods of inducing labor, such as eating spicy foods, taking a walk, or having sex, none are guaranteed or scientifically proven. But hey, no harm in having some fun before baby comes!

Just hang in there. You might feel tired and uncomfortable, but you're so close to holding your sweet baby. And after nine months, in the scheme of things, it's not long at all now.

Nursery Room Odds and Ends

Some of the items you'll receive for the nursery room will be for you as much as they are for your sweet baby. Place each nursery room item at the top with the person in the box at the bottom who will find it most useful. If the item will be helpful to both mom and baby, place it in the middle box.

Crib

Mattress

Rocking Chair

White Noise Machine

Nightlight

Wipes

Changing Pad

Baby Monitor

Diaper Pail

Diapers

Burp Cloth

Nursing Pillow

Pacifier

MOM	MOM AND BABY	BABY

Would You Rather?

Pregnancy and motherhood can sometimes force you to make some crazy choices. Circle the least cringeworthy option from each line.

1. Birth a baby **on a plane** or **in a car**?

2. Clean up **spit up** or a **diaper blowout**?

3. Have your water break **at work during a presentation** or **in a crowded restaurant on date night**?

4. Have a **dirty spit up blanket** or **soiled diaper in a hot car** for one week?

5. Give up **alcohol for a year** or **experience childbirth without drugs**?

6. Give up **your body pillow** or **your leggings** during your pregnancy?

7. Have **a bunch of strangers try to touch your belly** or **have a bunch of strangers offer you unsolicited parenting advice**?

8. Have **heartburn for nine months** or **hemorrhoids for nine months**?

9. Have **explosive diarrhea for a month** or **nonstop lactating breasts for a month**?

10. Have **two months of postpartum excessive hair loss** or **postpartum problematic acne**?

11. Have your baby's name chosen by **a stranger** or **your partner's mother**?

12. Carry baby weight in **your breasts** or **your butt**?

13. Have a **nice but inexperienced OB-GYN** or a **veteran doctor who calls you "big girl"**?

14. Have a partner who **faints during delivery** or a partner who **livestreams the entire thing**?

15. Grow hair **on your chin** or **belly** during pregnancy?

Childbirth MythBusters

Some of these old stories are true, but some are bunk. Do you know your folk wisdom from your fairy tales? Find out by answering True or False to the following questions.

Childbirth is like what you see on TV. T / F

Spicy food kick-starts labor. T / F

You have to give birth on your back. T / F

Eating vegetables while pregnant will help your baby like them later. T / F

Pregnancy heartburn means you'll give birth to a baby with more hair. T / F

An epidural may hinder your chances for breastfeeding success. T / F

You will know when you're in labor. T / F

Sex can kick-start contractions. T / F

Your birth plan is the perfect playbook for having your baby. T / F

SEVEN THINGS ABOUT CHILDBIRTH
THEY DON'T SHOW YOU IN THE MOVIES

You've probably seen a ton of movies and TV shows where pregnant women go into labor, but Hollywood doesn't tell you the whole story. Here are some kind of weird but totally normal things that might happen when you're giving birth:

Your water might not dramatically break.
There's always a huge gush of water that splashes all over the floor if you're a pregnant lady giving birth in a movie, but you're a real person, so you might actually start labor without a trickle. If that happens, the doctor will break your water for you. You might also start labor with your water breaking as a steady trickle that feels a little bit like you peed on yourself.

You'll feel like you need to poop.
When your baby has descended into position and is ready to come through the birth canal, you'll feel pressure everywhere down there. Really, everywhere. Your nurses know what that pressure means, though: It's time to push out your baby!

Still, you will probably poop.
It's VERY common to poop while you're pushing out baby. Do not think twice about it. Doctors and nurses have seen it a million times, and they won't make a big deal of it at all. In fact, you might not even know you did it!

You have to deliver the placenta.
Once your baby is out, your job isn't done yet. Contractions will continue for a bit while your uterus works to deliver the placenta. During this time, the doctor will make sure everything else is good and take care of any stitches you might need.

You might feel like vomiting.
You've spent a significant amount of time going through contractions and putting pressure on your insides. Depending on how your labor went, you might have also taken a bunch of medications. You might need to throw up. It's not unusual.

You're stronger than you think.
Labor is really, really hard. There will be times you might feel like you can't do it. But our bodies are powerful, and they are designed to do this! It might be a marathon, so take those breaths. Birth is an incredible thing, and once you go through it, you'll be amazed at how strong you really are.

Childhood Traditions

Think about the best parts of your childhood that you hope your baby gets to experience. Fill in each line with some of your fondest childhood memories or traditions you hope to carry on with your own growing family:

I spent holidays with _____

_____

_____

I celebrated my birthday by _____

_____

_____

My favorite gift was _____

_____

_____

During the summers, we _____

_____

_____

My favorite place to go was _____

_____

_____

The best thing about where we lived was _____

_____

_____

I Am New Mom, Hear Me Roar

Labor and delivery are hard enough . . . You don't have to be hard on yourself, too. In fact, it's the perfect time to be kind to yourself! Fill in each blank with a positive affirmation.

1. This is my story and no one else's. I am grateful that _____
_____

2. I am not alone. These are the people I can talk to for support: _____
_____

3. No one is judging me. My body is _____
_____

4. My body is doing exactly what it needs to be doing. I look _____
_____

5. My baby is _____
_____

6. I am _____ every day.

7. I am not perfect. But I am doing _____ really well.

8. I am a blessing to my child because _____
_____

9. Today, I will notice the positive aspects of motherhood, such as _____
_____

10. I am strong because _____
_____

Nursery Needs

Before you bring home your baby, you'll want to set up their little nursery.
This crossword puzzle reveals some of the equipment you'll need for your
newborn.

Across

3. Where diapers
   meet wipes
5. Short for fanatic
7. Poop catcher
10. Sound to
    block sounds
12. Gentle up and
    down chair
13. They usually
    come wet

Down

1. A little illumination
2. Wetness guard for
   nighttime
4. Now I lay me down
   to sleep
6. For rocking
   and feeding
8. Wicker box
   with no top
9. Gas release fabric
11. Comfy part of a bed

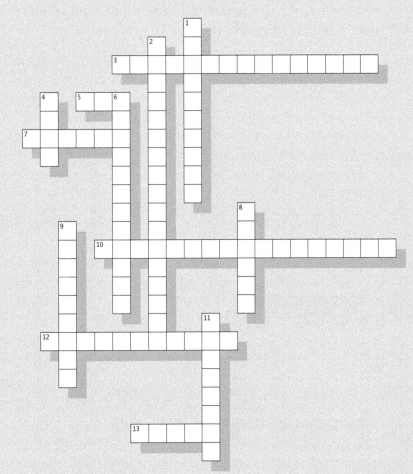

Swaddle the Baby

Dreams of your sweet swaddled baby can sometimes be interrupted, literally, as the sound of tears come crashing through. Here's the thing: Babies cry. It's how they express themselves, usually when they're hungry, cold, dirty, or overtired, or even when they have some unused energy to expend. Swaddling is a great way to calm your sweet babe, so it's important to learn how! Put these steps for swaddling in the correct order then draw them in empty boxes on the left side of the page.

STEP _____:
Pull the bottom of the blanket up and over the feet and toward your baby's shoulder, without making the legs too tight.

STEP _____:
Fold the corner snugly across your baby's chest and tuck it beneath baby.

STEP _____:
Arrange the blanket on a safe surface in a diamond shape, and fold the top corner down. Set your baby on top with shoulders at the fold.

STEP _____:
Pull one side of the blanket diagonally across your baby's chest and tuck it under baby's body.

Remembrance of Trimesters Past . . .

The end of your pregnancy is the perfect time to take a moment to reflect on your journey. Writing your memories down now will help them stay fresh, and it'll be such a joy to share with your child someday.

When I first found out I was pregnant, I immediately thought _____

_____

My nickname for my baby is _____

_____

My favorite thing about my pregnancy is _____

_____

I initially thought I was having a BOY/GIRL

When I found out the gender, I _____

_____

This pregnancy, I've been feeling _____

_____

I can't believe I ate so much _____

_____

Hearing my baby's heartbeat on the monitor felt _____

_____

I couldn't stand the smell of _____

_____

Hospital Room Fun

Spot the differences between the two rooms. Hint: There are 10 differences.

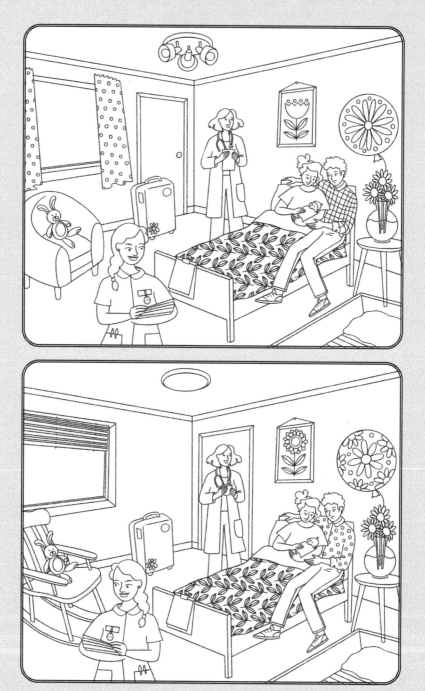

The Birth Canal Zone

Help the baby get delivered!

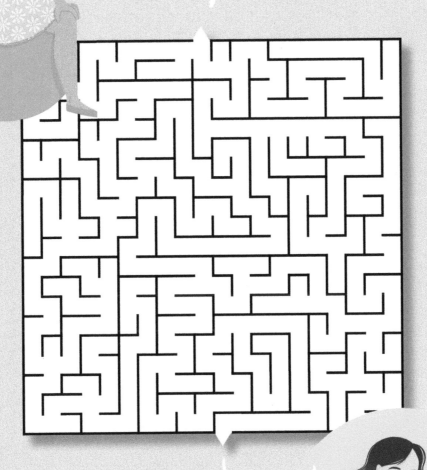

WHEN CAN I GO HOME?

When you have *some* idea of how long your hospital stay might last, it will help you pack your hospital bag, make plans for your pets, prepare for your return home, and get into the right frame of mind for being away from home. You can think of this as a mini holiday, probably with more pudding cups than you're used to!

While a hospital isn't necessarily a fun place to be, it's definitely a place where you are taken care of. Breakfast, lunch, and dinner will be brought to you in bed. Nurses are there to help change diapers and swaddle your baby. Doctors, nurses, and lactation consultants are nearby for any questions or issues. No matter what the length your hospital stay may be, try to enjoy it while you're there.

The length of stay depends on your insurance, your doctor, and the health of you and your baby. For a standard vaginal delivery with no complications, the usual discharge is between 24 and 48 hours. You'll need some time to rest and let any medication wear off. During that postpartum hospital stay, both you and your baby will be monitored to make sure no problems arise. As long as everyone is doing well, you can even talk to your doctor about an early discharge.

For a C-section with no complications, a hospital stay usually lasts between two and four days. Your doctor will want to make sure you can urinate, pass gas, get up and walk around, and eat and drink without vomiting. Usually you'll have to wait for a while before you can have any food after the surgery.

Check with your doctor, hospital, and insurance provider if you need a clearer idea of what to expect. Even though it's good to prepare mentally, you should know that truly, it all comes down to the delivery! Your medical team will determine together when you and your baby are ready to head home.

Mama's Choice

Think about your perfect childbirth experience, then circle your top choice from each line. A mom can dream (and a mom can make demands).

midwife **OR** doctor

hospital birth **OR** home birth

music **OR** silence

sandals **OR** slippers

medication-free **OR** medicated childbirth

ice chips **OR** ice pop

long labor **OR** long pushing

breast milk **OR** formula

early discharge **OR** extra night in the hospital

congratulatory note **OR** personal visit

flowers **OR** candy

postpartum sushi **OR** postpartum wine

Connecting with the Baby

Join the dots to reveal the picture.

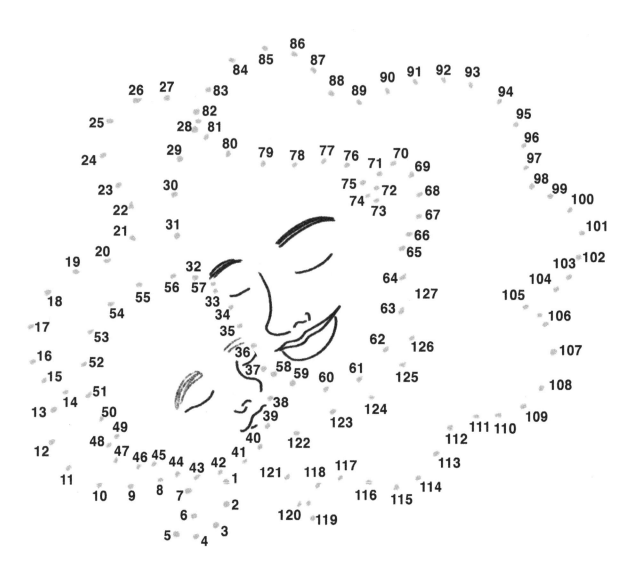

Parturition Paraphernalia

The labor and delivery room is no place for the faint of heart. But that room—and this word search—are places where you'll find all of the following things. Look for them in all directions, including backward and diagonally.

Doctor	Contraction	Breathing	Placenta
Nurse	Labor	Stirrups	Umbilical
Mom	Delivery	Dilation	Exhaustion
Baby	Monitor	Gown	Recovery
Push	Epidural	Scrubs	

```
E C Q L A T P T G O T U B N I U Y
Y O O A Z R H O K U N T R U I U C
U S S C S M J C O U U Z E R Y H O
Z R M I X O N P D P M P A S E C M
K C C L C M F O P Q C T T E X O M
G F D I Y P O N I D S A H C H N K
O N L B L R L N C T I I I X A T R
W I D M D M E A I G A E N T U R E
N U A U A O P V C T A L G F S A C
L A B O R P C T I E O R I D T C O
B R I T F S I T K L N R U D I T V
S B U R C S U N O R E T F E O I E
M E P I D U R A L R T D A A N O R
W A M Q J T X S W R O W J D Y N Y
P H S U P Y B A B S T I R R U P S
```

NICU

A mom never *wants* her baby to be in the NICU, the neonatal intensive care unit. But you may want to seek out a hospital with one of these intensive care nurseries, just in case a NICU stay is needed. If your baby does need to go, this special nursery will be filled with round-the-clock care from a team of experts.

The NICU is different from the regular newborn nursery, and some hospitals have both. It's good to ask your doctor ahead of time to find out where your baby will go should the need arise for special care. It's good to be informed ahead of time so that as changes arise, you can understand what's happening and make better choices.

There are a few reasons your baby could be admitted to the NICU. The NICU takes in premature babies and babies who have other health problems, including an infection or respiratory issues. Your baby may even go to the NICU for additional testing if you had a high-risk pregnancy. Once babies are breathing and eating on their own, it's usually time to be released. Of course, your baby's care team will keep you informed on your baby's progress.

Thankfully, parents can visit and spend time with their babies in the NICU. Often mothers can hold and feed their little ones as well. In fact, touch and skin-to-skin contact is the best kind of bonding and care for your child.

If your baby does end up in the NICU, you have to remember to take care of YOU. Find ways to reduce stress, pay attention to your own needs, get the nourishment your body needs, try to sleep, and talk to someone. A NICU stay can be a difficult thing to adjust to, but you can take comfort in knowing that your baby is getting the best kind of care.

What Does Not Belong?

Circle the one item from each section that does NOT belong.

1. HOSPITAL

doctor, baby toys, ice chips

2. BIRTHING ROOM

monitor, speculum, bottle warmer

3. NURSERY

crib, changing pad, laundry soap

4. CAR

car seat, play mat, diaper bag

5. HOSPITAL BAG

slippers, lip balm, jeans

6. DIAPER BAG

diapers, mobile, pacifier

Pregnancy Superlatives

Fill in the blank with your favorite things about pregnancy.

Biggest craving _____

Best compliment _____

Most enjoyable _____

Most surprising _____

Most exciting _____

Most tiring _____

Most hours slept _____

Most humiliating _____

Most painful _____

Most thought about _____

Most comical _____

Most talked about _____

Most complicated _____

Most tears over _____

Most watched _____

Most said during labor _____

Most precious moment _____

Time to Meet Your Baby!

Fill in the blanks with the correct answers so you can remember the details later. This way your child can't accuse you of exaggerating when you tell them the story of their birth!

The time of the first contraction was _

_____

We arrived at the hospital at _____

_____

My water broke at _____

_____

I spent _____hours in labor

I pushed _____ times

The people in the room during labor

were _____

The baby weighed _____

The baby was _____ inches

The baby was born in the city of _____

_____

The baby was born at _____

_____ a.m./p.m.

My favorite moment during labor was

_____

The person who caught the baby was .

_____

The time of the baby's first feeding

was _____

The first diaper change happened at _

_____

The first bath happened at _____

_____

What's Missing Now?

Once your baby is here, your new obsession may be keeping a close eye on every move they make—every eye and neck movement, facial expression, and arm wave. But keeping track of miscellaneous and replaceable items? Not so much. In this picture, see if you can locate the most common misplaced baby items: a pacifier, a baby shoe, a blanket, a stuffed teddy bear, and a bottle.

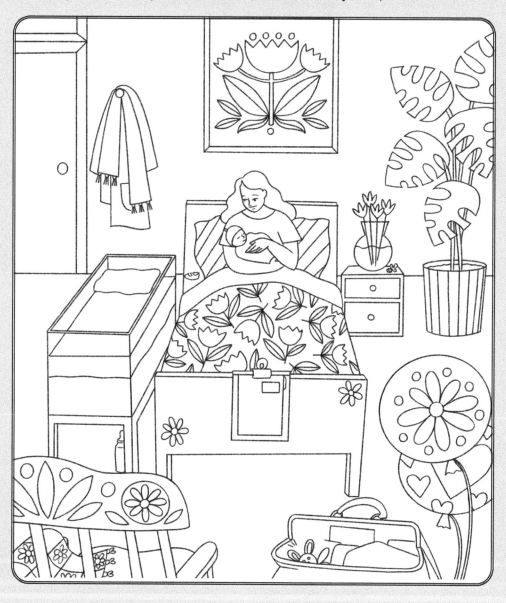

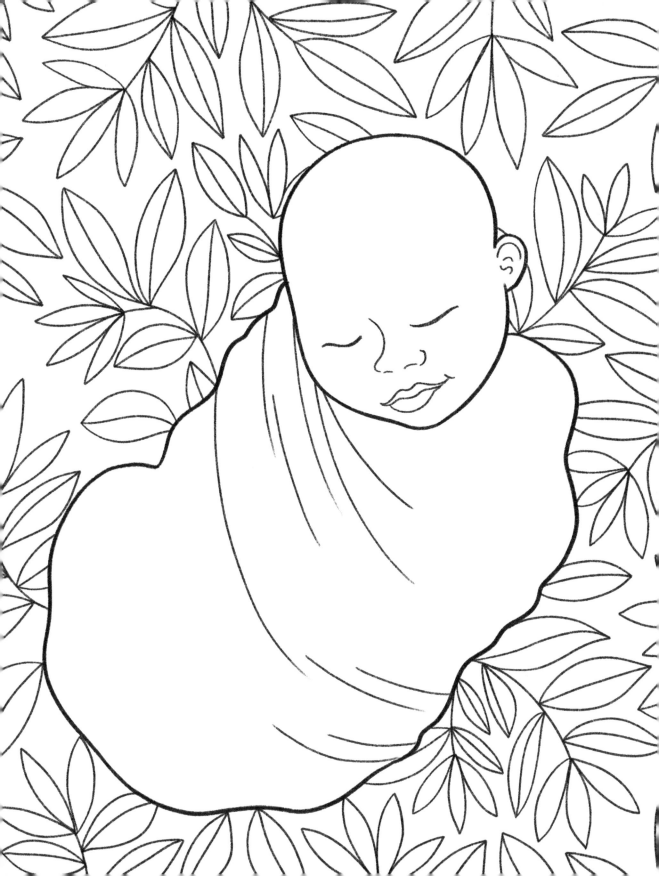

Resources

FRESHMOMMYBLOG.COM. Stay connected with me and find additional motherhood and lifestyle tips on the site! From postpartum care to living your best life as a family, my aim is to empower your motherhood journey.

BABYCENTER.COM. A site filled with tips from pregnancy to child development. There's even an app you can download to track each week of your pregnancy and what's happening in your body.

THE FIRST FORTY DAYS: The Essential Art of Nourishing the New Mother by Heng Ou. This book provides a wealth of information on recovering postpartum and allows you to better understand and appreciate what has happened in your body. It also teaches how to nourish yourself during the unofficial "fourth trimester" that is postpartum.

References

"6 Surprising Facts About Your Pregnant Body." Parents. Accessed December 18, 2019. www.parents.com/pregnancy/my-body/changing/6-surprising-facts -about-your-pregnant-body/.

"10 Old Wives' Tales About Pregnancy: What's True And What's Not?" Care. com. January 8, 2020. www.care.com/c/stories/4929/10-best-pregnancy-old -wives-tales/.

American Pregnancy Association. "Dizziness During Pregnancy." Accessed November 8, 2019. americanpregnancy.org/pregnancy-health /dizziness -during-pregnancy/.

American Academy of Family Physicians. "Your Baby's Development: The First Trimester." Accessed October 2016. familydoctor.org/your-babys-development -the-first-trimester

American Academy of Family Physicians. "Your Baby's Development: The Second Trimester." Accessed October 2016. familydoctor.org/your-babys -development-the-second-trimester

American Academy of Family Physicians. "Your Baby's Development: The Third Trimester." Accessed October 2016. familydoctor.org/your-babys-development -the-third-trimester

Blue, Tabitha. "My Birth Story Changed Fast When I Developed Preeclampsia During Pregnancy." BabyCenter. May 1, 2018. www.babycenter.com /0_preeclampsia_257.bc.

Ben-Joseph, Elana Pearl, ed. "Can Pregnant Women Do Anything to Reduce or Prevent Swollen Ankles? (for Parents) - Nemours KidsHealth." The Nemours Foundation, July 2015. kidshealth.org/en/parents/ankles.html.

Cadle, C. Joseph. "Shortness of Breath During Pregnancy." TheBump.com - Pregnancy, Parenting and Baby Information. The Bump, August 19, 2014. www.thebump.com/a/shortness-of-breath-during-pregnancy.

Centers for Disease Control and Prevention. "Recommendations: Women & Folic Acid." Accessed December 13, 2019. www.cdc.gov/ncbddd/folicacid /recommendations.html

De Pietro, MaryAnn, CRT. "Second Trimester Pains: What to Expect." Medical News Today. www.medicalnewstoday.com/articles/323799.php#causes.

"Fetal Development: What Happens during the 2nd Trimester?" Mayo Clinic. Mayo Foundation for Medical Education and Research, July 8, 2017. www.mayoclinic.org/healthy-lifestyle/pregnancy-week-by-week/in-depth /fetal-development/art-20046151?pg=1.

"Fetal Development: What Happens during the 3rd Trimester?" Mayo Clinic. Mayo Foundation for Medical Education and Research, July 6, 2017. www.mayoclinic.org/healthy-lifestyle/pregnancy-week-by-week/in-depth /fetal-development/art-20045997.

Frank, Christina, and Elizabeth Stein. "What to Expect After Giving Birth in a Hospital." Parents. Accessed December 19, 2019. www.parents.com/pregnancy /giving-birth/labor-and-delivery/qa-what-can-i-expect-in-the-delivery-room -after-ive-given/.

Hytten, F. 1985. "Blood Volume Changes in Normal Pregnancy." Clinics in Haematology. U.S. National Library of Medicine. October 1985. www.ncbi.nlm .nih.gov/pubmed/4075604.

"Is It Normal to Have Weird Dreams during Pregnancy?" n.d. Parents. Accessed December 19, 2019. www.parents.com/pregnancy/my-body/is-it-normal-to -have-weird-dreams-during-pregnancy/.

Johnson, Traci C. "Get the Calcium You Need During Pregnancy." Health & Baby Medical Reference, WebMD. Accessed December 13, 2018. webmd.com /baby/get-the-calcium-you-need-during-pregnancy#1

Johnson, Traci C. "Leg Cramps During Pregnancy: How To Stop & Prevent Them." WebMD. WebMD, July 2, 2018. www.webmd.com/baby/leg-cramps.

Johnson, Traci C. "Tests You Might Receive in 3rd Trimester of Pregnancy." WebMD. WebMD, September 9, 2018. www.webmd.com/baby/guide/third -trimester-tests.

Johnson, Traci C. and Trina Pagano. "Pregnancy Visual Timeline." Health and Pregnancy Center, WebMD. Accessed December 13, 2019. webmd.com/baby/interactive-pregnancy-tool-fetal-development?week=2

Kandola, Aaron. "Braxton-Hicks vs. Real Contractions: Differences and Signs." Medical News Today. MediLexicon International, January 30, 2019. www.medicalnewstoday.com/articles/324326.php.

Lee, Megan, and Joanne Bradbury. "Five Types of Food to Increase Your Psychological Well-Being." Medical Xpress - medical research advances and health news. Medical Xpress, September 10, 2018. medicalxpress.com/news/2018-09-food-psychological-well-being.html.

Marple, Katie. "Fetal Development Week by Week." BabyCenter. Accessed December 13, 2019. babycenter.com/fetal-development-week-by-week

"Medicine: Prodigious Pregnancy." Time. Time Inc., March 5, 1945. http://content.time.com/time/magazine/article/0,9171,797153,00.html.

Nierenberg, Cari. "Mood Swings & Mommy Brain: The Emotional Challenges of Pregnancy." LiveScience. Purch, December 22, 2017. www.livescience.com/51043-pregnancy-emotions.html.

"Pregnancy Advice: Old Wives Tales Vs. Science." n.d. Parents. Accessed December 23, 2019. www.parents.com/pregnancy/my-body/pregnancy-health/pregnancy-advice-old-wives-vs-science/.

"Pregnancy Emotions." American Pregnancy Association, October 16, 2019. americanpregnancy.org/pregnancy-concerns/pregnancy-emotions/.

"Pregnancy and Heartburn." Stanford Children's Health - Lucile Packard Children's Hospital Stanford. Accessed December 19, 2019. www.stanfordchildrens.org/en/topic/default?id=pregnancy-and-heartburn-134-10.

"Pregnancy & Sleep." National Sleep Foundation. Accessed December 19, 2019. www.sleepfoundation.org/articles/pregnancy-and-sleep.

"Prenatal Care: 1st Trimester Visits." Mayo Clinic. Mayo Foundation for Medical Education and Research, November 10, 2018. www.mayoclinic.org/healthy-lifestyle/pregnancy-week-by-week/in-depth/prenatal-care/art-20044882.

Saftlas, Audrey F, Elizabeth W Triche, Hind Beydoun, and Michael B Bracken. 2010. "Does Chocolate Intake during Pregnancy Reduce the Risks of Preeclampsia and Gestational Hypertension?" Annals of Epidemiology. U.S. National Library of Medicine. August 2010. www.ncbi.nlm.nih.gov/pmc /articles/PMC2901253/.

Staff, Familydoctor.org Editorial. "Your Baby's Development: The Second Trimester." familydoctor.org, January 25, 2018. familydoctor.org/your-babys -development-the-second-trimester/.

Staff, Familydoctor.org Editorial. "Sleep and Pregnancy." familydoctor.org, June 6, 2017. familydoctor.org/getting-enough-sleep-pregnancy/.

Spears, Nina. "What To Do In Early Labor." Baby Chick, February 5, 2019. www.babychick.com/what-to-do-in-early-labor/.

The American College of Obstetricians and Gynecologists. "Exercise During Pregnancy." Accessed December 13, 2019. acog.org/patient resources/faqs /pregnancy/exercise-during-pregnancy

The American College of Obstetricians and Gynecologists. "Nutrition During Pregnancy." Accessed December 13, 2019. acog.org/patient-resources/faqs /pregnancy/nutrition-during-pregnancy

The American Pregnancy Association. "Pregnancy Week 12." Accessed December 13, 2019. www.americanpregnancy.org/week-by-week/12 -weeks-pregnant

The University of Chicago Medicine. "Tips to Manage Common Pregnancy Symptoms by Trimester." Accessed December 14, 2019. www.uchicagomedicine .org/forefront/womens-health-articles/tips-to-manage-common-pregnancy -symptoms-by-trimester.

Todd, Nivin. "Braxton Hicks: Definition, What They Feel Like, and Triggers." WebMD. WebMD, March 2, 2020. www.webmd.com/baby/guide/true-false-labor#2.

Timmons, Jessica. "Insomnia in Early Pregnancy: Why It Happens and What to Do." Healthline. Healthline Media, January 6, 2020. www.healthline.com/health /pregnancy/early-insomnia.

"Using Epidural Anesthesia During Labor: Benefits and Risks." American Pregnancy Association, October 13, 2019. americanpregnancy.org/labor -and-birth/epidural/.

You and Your Hormones. "Relaxin." Accessed December 13, 2019. November 26, 2018. Accessed December 14, 2019. www.yourhormones.info/hormones/relaxin

"Your Baby's Development: The Second Trimester." Familydoctor.org. January 25, 2018. familydoctor.org/your-babys-development-the-second-trimester/.

Index

Answer Key

First Trimester

Amazing Mama

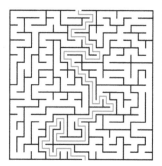

Gestation Indications

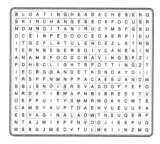

Foods to Avoid

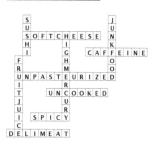

Pregnancy Exercises Quiz

1. A.
2. True
3. D.
4. D.
5. B.
6. C.
7. C.
8. False
9. B.
10. B.
11. D.

First Trimester Firsts

kick

ultrasound

doctor

heartbeat

nausea

fetus

craving

hormones

tired

morning sickness

mood swings

weight gain

prenatal

genetic tests

baby names

saltines

test

twelve weeks

aversion

First Trimester Quiz

1. A.
2. True
3. C.
4. C.
5. A.
6. D.
7. D.
8. D.
9. D.
10. D.
11. True
12. A.
13. True
14. C.

Out of Order

1 week: Period

2 weeks: Ovulation

3 weeks: Fertilization

4 weeks: Implantation

5 weeks: Baby's heart begins to form

6 weeks: Buds appear that will become arms

7 weeks: Head develops

8 weeks: Fingers begin to form

9 weeks: Toes start to form

10 weeks: Elbows can bend

11 weeks: Genitals start to form

12 weeks: Finger-nails form

Second Trimester

What to Expect When You're Expanding

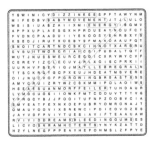

Pregnancy Needs

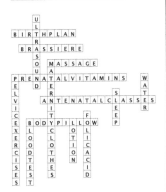

Registry Necessities Scramble

baby bottles

pacifier

wipes

onesies

breast pump

bibs

body pillow

baby monitor

diaper bag

stroller

car seat

high chair

diapers

nipple cream

bottle brush

burp cloths

crib

crib mattress

blankets

Pregnancy Aches and Pains

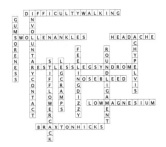

Bumped into New Symptoms

leg cramps

bigger belly

glucose test

back ache

water retention

dizziness

muscle spasms

increased food cravings

vivid dreams

heartburn

bleeding gums

waddle walk

clothes not fitting

tender breasts

linea negra

Getting through the Hump

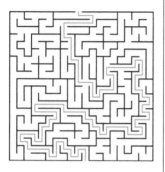

Pregnancy Dos and Don'ts

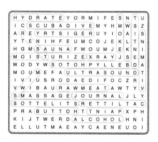

What's in a Pregnancy?

ace
age
ane
any
ape
arc
are
aye
can
cap
car
cay

cep
cry
ear
eng
era
erg
ern
gae
gan
gap
gar
gay
gen
gey
gyp
nae
nag
nan
nap
nay
neg
pac
pan
par
pay
pea
pec
peg
pen
per
pry
pya
pye
rag
ran
rap

ray
rec
reg
rep
rya
rye
yag
yap
yar
yea
yen
yep

Preeclampsia

1. True
2. True
3. True
4. False
5. True
6. False
7. True
8. True
9. False
10. True
11. True
12. False
13. False
14. True

What's Going On in There?

1. D.
2. C.
3. B.
4. B.
5. A.
6. C.
7. True
8. D.
9. D.

10. C.
11. B.
12. A.

Third Trimester

Mama's Little Self-Helper

stay positive
breakfast in bed
yoga poses
chocolate bar
warm milk
bubble bath
babymoon
power nap
relaxing music
journal entry

10 Things Baby Doesn't Need

baby towels
baby robe
wipes warmer
baby oil
boogie wipes
pacifier wipes
stuffed animals
newborn shoes
bath thermometer
bottle warmer

Get the Pregnant Woman to the Bathroom

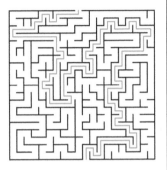

Gravely Tired

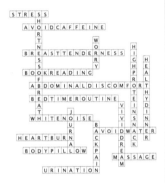

Big Belly Blues

vivid dreams
back pain
abdominal discomfort
frequent urination
leg cramps
shortness of breath
stress
heartburn
worry
varicose veins
fatigue

hemorrhoids
swollen ankles
insomnia

Maternal Instinct

airmen
attire
enmity
entity
etamin
imaret
inmate
marine
marten
martin
matier
matter
mattin
minter
mitten
natter
nitery
ratine
ratite
ratten
remain
remint
retain
retina
retint
tamein
tetany
tinter
titman
titmen
treaty

tyrant *(continued)*

yatter

yttria

Heartburn Help

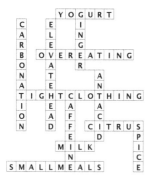

Pregnancy Relief from A to Z

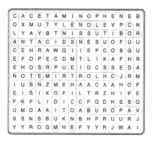

Nursery Essentials

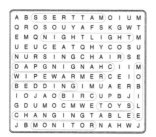

Nesting Checklist

install carseat

wash baby clothes

pack hospital bag

build crib

freeze meals

wash windows

sleep

wipe baseboards

declutter

schedule bills

wash bedding

clean carpets

dust fans

Delivery Room Match

MOM

Slippers

Robe

Contractions

Glow

Holding baby

NURSE

Cup of ice

Extra pillow

Wheelchair

Blankets

Meals

Pain medications

BABY

Diaper

Pacifier

Onesie

Mittens

Hat

Swaddle

PHOTOGRAPHER

Camera

Tripod

Flash

Pose

**OB-GYN/RESI-
DENT DOCTOR**

Prescription pad

Amniotic hook

Forceps

Scissors

Speculum

Sutures

Who's Your Baby?

1. C.
2. A.
3. C.
4. B.
5. A.
6. A.
7. C.
8. D.
9. True
10. D.

Registry Checklist

Tub

Wash

Lotion

Crib sheets

Pajamas

Socks

Onesies

Blankets

Swaddlers

Burp cloths

Bibs

Sleep sacks

Diaper pail

Diapers

Wipes

Diaper cream

Breast pump

Crib mattress

Nursing pillow

Bottles

High chair

Nail trimmer

Thermometer

Crib

Rocking chair

Changing table

Baby monitor

Bouncer

Teether

Car seat

Stroller

Baby carrier

Diaper bag

Play yard

The Waddle Workout

Tying shoelaces

Rolling over

Standing up

Walking

Climbing stairs

Breathing

Zipping pants

Shaving legs

Eating

Painting toenails

Talking

Childbirth

Baby Talk

1. C.
2. D.
3. A.
4. B.
5. C.
6. D.
7. A.
8. C.
9. D.
10. A.

Bring Baby Home!

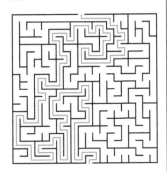

Baby's First Stuff

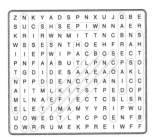

Mama Match

1. Thrust
2. Tightening
3. Pulsation
4. Liquid
5. Birth class
6. Physician
7. Caretaker
8. Howl
9. Bliss
10. Wrap
11. Childbirth
12. Infirmary

Expanding CONTRACTIONS

acrostic

actinons

arnottos

canonist

cantoris

carotins

cartoons

citators

coaction

coactors

conation

constant

contacts

contains

contorts

contract

contrast

cooncans

corantos

cortinas

cratonic

crostino *(continued)*

intrants

narcotic

nonactor

notation

notators

notornis

occasion

orations

oscitant

ostinato

ostracon

raccoons

rattoons

ricottas

rotation

sanction

sonantic

sonorant

strontia

strontic

tactions

tortonis

traction

Go-Bag Go-Time

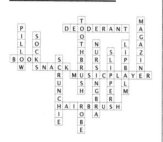

Delivering from DELIVERY

delver

derive

direly

drivel

eerily

eviler

eyelid

levied

levier

lieder

liever

livery

livyer

reived

relied

relive

revile

ridley

veiled

veiler

verily

Nursery Room Odds and Ends

MOM

Nightlight

Baby Monitor

Burp Cloth

Diaper Pail

MOM AND BABY

Rocking Chair

Nursing Pillow

Pacifier

BABY

Crib

Mattress

Changing Pad

White Noise Machine

Wipes

Diapers

Childbirth MythBusters

False

False

False

True

True

False

False

True

False

Nursery Needs

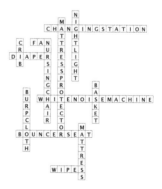

Swaddle the Baby

STEP 1: Arrange the blanket on a safe surface in a diamond shape, and fold the top corner down. Set your baby on top with shoulders at the fold.

STEP 2: Pull one side of the blanket diagonally across your baby's chest and tuck it under baby's body.

STEP 3: Pull the bottom of the blanket up and over the feet and toward your baby's shoulder, without making the legs too tight.

STEP 4: Fold the last corner snugly across your baby's chest and tuck it beneath baby.

Hospital Room Fun

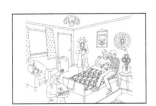

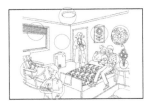

Differences:

Words on balloons

Pictures on the wall

Pattern on dad's shirt

Items the doctor is holding

Hat on baby's head in one photo

Direction the nurse is facing

Where the door is located

Curtains vs. no curtains

Ceiling lights are different

Rocking chair vs. regular chair

The Birth Canal Zone

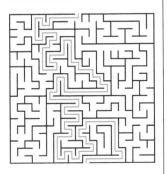

Parturition Paraphernalia

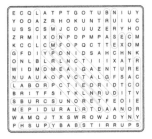

What Does Not Belong?

1. Hospital - baby toys
2. Birthing Room - speculum
3. Nursery - laundry soap
4. Car - play mat
5. Hospital bag - jeans
6. Diaper bag - mobile

What's Missing Now?

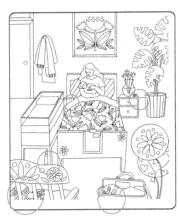

Acknowledgments

First, I want to show my utmost gratitude for the many families and mamas who've come alongside and supported our family adventures and the words we share with our online community. It's because of you I realize that all of us mothers need to know we're not alone, especially during pregnancy. It's been a privilege to share our lives with you, and I'm grateful that we can bring some lighthearted fun, with a bit of encouragement, to new mamas through these pages.

To the team at Callisto Media: The whole team has been amazing to work with throughout the process. Especially Vanessa Putt for bringing me on board with such a fun project and Shannon Criss for her expertise and support as we navigated each page.

To my family: It is only because of you that I'm inspired to write and share parts of our journey with other moms. I remember all of those "firsts" with each of you and want to make each "first" for other moms be just as magical, if not moreso. Thank you for being my inspiration.

To my husband: Chris, those late nights sitting at the dining room table and helping me come up with clues for words like diaper and breast tenderness . . . Thank you for being there, for making me laugh, for encouraging me through the process both of having our own babies and of birthing this book. I wouldn't have done it without you.

About the Author

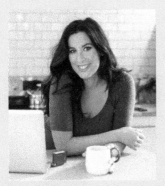

TABITHA BLUE is a certified life coach and founder of *Fresh Mommy Blog*, which captures the journey of her family's lives and travels and her attempt at domesticity. This supportive and creative online community has grown right along with her family of eight. After years of blogging on motherhood, *Fresh Mommy Blog* relaunched in 2017 as a full lifestyle brand—a space where thousands come for tips and tricks on everything from home design to DIY projects, delicious recipes, fashion and style inspiration, and of course fun stories and life lessons. Tabitha is also the host of House to Home, a DIY home renovation series on YouTube, and editor of *The Fresh Edit*, a lifestyle magazine.

CPSIA information can be obtained
at www.ICGtesting.com
Printed in the USA
JSHW011055080421
13244JS00002B/3